Antonia Deiza Rodrigues de Carvalho
CamilaSabrina Oliveira Lima
Luisa Helena Oliveira Lima

Breastfeeding in the First Hour of Life

Antonia Deiza Rodrigues de Carvalho
CamilaSabrina Oliveira Lima
Luisa Helena Oliveira Lima

Breastfeeding in the First Hour of Life

Influence of obstetric variables

Table of contents:

Antonia Deiza Rodrigues de Carvalho

Camila Sabrina de Oliveira Lima

Luisa Helena de Oliveira Lima

BREASTFEEDING IN THE FIRST HOUR OF LIFE Influence of obstetric variables

New Academic Editions

ACKNOWLEDGMENTS

Almost five years have passed and another stage has been completed in my life. Now the goals and expectations for new achievements have changed. Knowledge has been acquired and challenges have been overcome, but alone it would be impossible to count this victory.

First of all, I thank **GOD**, for giving me the strength and resignation to get through all the obstacles, tiredness and discouragement, if it hadn't been for his outstretched hands to help me, I probably wouldn't have reached my ultimate goal, to "Him be all honor and glory".

To my parents, **FRANCISCA AND FRANCISCO**, "who gave me life" and taught me how to live it with dignity, who illuminated the dark paths with affection and a lot of dedication so that I could walk without fear and full of hope. Mom, it was your care and dedication that gave me the strength to go on at times. Dad, your presence has meant security and the certainty that I am not alone on this journey. I can't thank you enough, I LOVE YOU!

To my sisters, **DENISE, DAYANE AND DARTICLÉIA,** thank you for your patience, encouragement and companionship, and for always supporting me with words and gestures along the way, you are angels in my life, I LOVE YOU.

To the rest of my family, my grandparents, godparents, brothers-in-law, nephews, uncles and aunts, cousins, you were also essential in my journey, thank you for always rooting for me and for my happiness.

To my old friends, for understanding my moments of absence. I would especially like to thank my "little sister" Rosane, who, even at a distance, is always by my side, supporting me and giving me a tug when necessary.

To my new friends that I made during my years at university, thank you for the great times I was able to share with you. I'm especially grateful to Gabrielly and Maila, you were great allies on this long journey, one always supporting the other in times of difficulty, which weren't few, right? We are that duo of three, Trio Parada Dura, that I will always carry in my heart.

To my advisor, Professor Dr. Luisa Helena, for all her teachings, dedication and patience. Thank you for giving me the opportunity to take part in the Children's Health Research Group.

To my boyfriend, Eduardo Saraiva, for being such a wonderful person, who is always by my side, supporting me and encouraging me to be a better person every day, thank you for everything, my beautiful.

To everyone who directly or indirectly encouraged me not to give up and contributed to the realization of this dream, THANK YOU!

SUMMARY

Breastfeeding in the first hour of life after childbirth brings countless benefits to the mother-child binomial and is a fundamental factor in the nutritional, motor, cognitive and psychosocial development of the newborn. The aim of this study was to analyze the influence of obstetric and socioeconomic variables on the development of breastfeeding in the first hour of life. This is a descriptive, cross-sectional study with a quantitative approach, carried out in a public reference hospital in the municipality of Picos-PI, by 587 mothers whose children were born alive between January and December 2015. The results showed that the prevalence of breastfeeding in the first hour of life occurred in almost two-thirds of mothers, and was 90% higher among women who gave birth vaginally compared to those who had a caesarean section. The fact that the women lived in rural areas increased the chances of their newborn being breastfed in the first hour of life by 70% compared to those living in urban areas. The results suggest that factors related to childbirth care and living conditions have the greatest influence on the timely initiation of breastfeeding.

Keywords: Breastfeeding. Mother-child relationship. Maternal and child health. Nursing. Childbirth.

Chapter 1

1 INTRODUCTION

Breastfeeding brings countless benefits to the mother-child binomial and is a fundamental factor in the nutritional, motor, cognitive and psychosocial development of the newborn (NB), especially when it takes place in the first hour of life after birth.

Breast milk has a balanced composition of essential nutrients for the growth and development of the NB and is adapted to the child's metabolism. The World Health Organization (WHO) recommends Exclusive Breastfeeding (EBF) for the first six months of life, as it is sufficient to meet the baby's nutritional needs (RODRIGUES *et al.*, 2013).

Breastfeeding should be started within the first hour of life, in the delivery room, if the mother and newborn are in good health. Breastfeeding in the First Hour of Life (BFHI) corresponds to step four of the Baby-Friendly Hospital Initiative (BFHI), and is part of a public policy to promote breastfeeding and reduce infant mortality. Step four of the BFHI recommends: "placing babies in direct contact with their mothers immediately after birth for at least one hour and encouraging mothers to identify when their babies are ready to breastfeed, providing help if necessary (BOCCOLINI *et al.*, 2013; POSSOLLI *et al.*, 2015).

APHV is considered to be an indicator of excellence in breastfeeding. In this sense, the WHO classifies the percentage of adherence to breastfeeding in the first hour for healthy mothers and newborns between 0 and 29% as "very bad", 30 to 49% "bad", 50 to 89% "good" and 90 to 100% "very good" (BELO *et al.*, 2014).

According to Carvalho *et al* (2016), the prevalence of APHV among babies born in Brazil in 2011-2012 was 56%, which represents an improvement on the 43% found in the National Demographic and Health Survey (PNDS) in 2006 (PNDS, 2006). However, the results were lower than those found in a study carried out in 2008 in Brazilian state capitals, where 67% of babies were breastfed within the first hour after birth (BRASIL, 2009). A systematic review of the literature by Esteves *et al* (2014) showed that APHV varied from 11.4% in one province in Saudi Arabia to 83.3% in Sri Lanka.

Studies have proven the countless benefits that APHV brings to the mother-child binomial: children who are breastfed soon after birth have a direct impact on a longer duration of breastfeeding and total breastfeeding; it promotes a greater emotional bond between mother and child; babies cry less; skin-to-skin contact keeps the NB at an adequate temperature, preventing hypothermia; breastfeeding stimulates the production of oxytocin, a hormone that causes the uterus to contract and involute, reducing the risks of uterine atony, hemorrhage and postpartum anemia (SÁ, 2015; VILLACA *et al.*, 2015; LEITE *et al.*, 2016).

Breast milk, especially colostrum, which is the milk secreted in the first few days postpartum, contains various protective factors (antibodies, vitamins, maturation factors, among others), which prevent the NB from infections, especially respiratory and gastrointestinal infections, physiological jaundice and hypoglycemia, thus reducing neonatal mortality rates and early hospitalizations (NUNES, 2015).

Although the importance of APHV has already been demonstrated, there are some obstetric variables that prevent or delay early breastfeeding, including absence of prenatal care (PN) appointments; lack of guidance on breastfeeding during PN follow-up; low level of maternal schooling; primiparous and/or adolescent women; mothers who are Human Immunodeficiency Virus (HIV) positive; lack of support for mothers in the delivery room; maternal anxiety; discomfort and discomfort during the first breastfeeding contacts; insufficient volumes of breast milk and/or delayed milk letdown; and caesarean section (ESTEVES *et al.*, 2015; V1LLACA *et al.*, 2015; SÁ, 2015; AGUAYO *et al.,* 2011).

According to Leite *et al* (2016), nursing's commitment becomes a determining factor in guaranteeing mothers and newborns the right to early breastfeeding, as its potential to promote health and reduce maternal and infant morbidity and mortality should be considered a priority when defining public policies aimed at women's and children's health. This makes it necessary to invest in programs that promote breastfeeding that is initiated and encouraged in the delivery room (ESTEVES *et al.*, 2015).

Considering that breastfeeding in the first hour of life is of great importance for the health of the child and the woman, this study asked: what obstetric variables influence the development of breastfeeding in the first hour of life?

The research is justified by the great importance of knowing the factors that influence the development of APHV in children from Pico, as well as expanding and seeking to rescue human care at the time of birth, seeking to reflect and question the actions and behaviors of the subjects involved in this process, since early breastfeeding is a practice of great importance for promoting and maintaining the health of the mother-child binomial.

In this way, the study seeks to contribute to highlighting the APHV; to add subsidies to improve the quality of the work of health professionals, preparing them to offer holistic, effective, supportive and integrative care; and to encourage health and education services to develop actions aimed at promoting effective and lasting MH and, consequently, a better quality of life for mothers and children.

Chapter 2

2 OBJECTIVES

2.1 General:

To analyze the influence of obstetric and socioeconomic variables on the development of breastfeeding in the first hour of life in newborns in Picos - PI.

2.2 Specific:

- The socio-economic and clinical profile of the mothers surveyed;
- To identify the prevalence of breastfeeding in the first hour of life in the population studied;
- To investigate the relationship between socio-economic variables and the development of breastfeeding in the first hour of life in children from Pico; and
- To verify the influence of prenatal care, guidance on breastfeeding, problems during pregnancy/partum/postpartum, and the type of delivery on the development of breastfeeding in the first hour of life in children from Pico.

Chapter 3

3 LITERATURE REVIEW

3.1 A brief history of breastfeeding

Breast milk has been recognized and recommended since biblical times as the ideal way to feed children in the first months of life. The period up to the 18th century has been poorly documented in terms of infant feeding, but it is known from records in private diaries that women breastfed their children during the 16th century. Until the 16th and 17th centuries, the breastfeeding of the Brazilian Tupinambás tribes had not been influenced by Europeans, but with colonization, the Portuguese brought the habit of using wet nurses, and this role was performed by black slaves (GRANJA; CUNHA, 2011).

In the second half of the 18th century, with the advent of the Industrial Revolution, the entry of women into the labor market and the increasing application of technological processes in the manufacture of food products, there were important stimuli for the development of artificial foods for infant feeding. In 1938, it was discovered that cow's milk was richer in protein than human milk, as well as the discovery of condensed milk, the evaporation of goat's milk and the study of the composition of human milk, which favored the production of artificial milk. (CAMINHA *et al.*, 2010).

Due to the great discouragement of breastfeeding, the state launched a major project at the end of the 19th century, "Puericulture", whose central theme was the feeding of children in general, with an emphasis on breastfeeding, beginning the process of "expropriation of popular knowledge about infant feeding by medical sciences." In 1978, the English doctor Underwood made the first recommendation to replace human milk with cow's milk. As a result, infant mortality rates rose in Europe (CAMINHA *et al.*, 2010; GRANJA; CUNHA, 2011).

At the beginning of the 20th century, birth and delivery were institutionalized, with the introduction of routines that contributed to the separation of mother and child and made it difficult to start breastfeeding, leading to the early weaning of children. At the same time, American industries were excelling in the production of human milk substitutes, discouraging breastfeeding. Faced with this reality, a nationwide campaign was launched in 1980 to sensitize politicians, health authorities, the media and community leaders to act in favor of breastfeeding, which led to the creation of various programs, policies and courses aimed at promoting, protecting and supporting early breastfeeding (MONTEIRO; NAKANO; GOMES, 2011).

In 1989, the WHO and the United Nations Children's Fund published a joint declaration entitled "Protecting, Promoting and Supporting Breastfeeding: The Special Role of Maternal and Child Health Services", whose main objectives were to disseminate the fundamental role that health services play in promoting and protecting breastfeeding and to describe what measures and actions should be taken to provide adequate information and support for mothers to practice breastfeeding. The ten steps to successful breastfeeding were proposed as an alternative to increase the prevalence and duration of breastfeeding in countries, with the fourth step being the APHV. In 2015, the APHV was included in the Global Reference List, which contains the 100 key indicators for monitoring health at national and global level (SÁ, 2015).

3.2 Programs to encourage breastfeeding in the first hour of life.

In order to encourage early breastfeeding, various programs and policies have been created in favor of the practice of breastfeeding, among them: the National Program to Encourage Breastfeeding (1981), the body responsible for coordinating policies in favor of breastfeeding; the Ordinance on Joint Lodging (1981); the implementation of the Network of Human Milk Banks (1985); the amendment to the Brazilian Constitution, extending maternity leave to 120 days (1988); the implementation of the Baby-Friendly Hospital Initiative (1992) and the commemoration of World Breastfeeding Week (1992) (MONTEIRO; NAKANO; GOMES, 2011).

Some courses were also created, such as the Counseling Course for Health Professionals and Awareness Raising for Managers (1996); the Counseling Course on Complementary Feeding for HIV Positive Mothers (1996); the Galba de Araújo Award (1999); the Breastfeeding Friendly Basic Unit Initiative (1999); and the Amamenta e Alimenta Brasil Network (2008) (MONTEIRO; NAKANO; GOMES, 2011).

■ Human Milk Banks

The Brazilian network of Human Milk Banks (BLH) was created in 1998, by a joint initiative of the Ministry of Health (MS) and the Oswaldo Cruz Foundation, with the aim of promoting, protecting and supporting breastfeeding; collecting and distributing human milk of certified quality; and contributing to reducing infant mortality (VILLAQA; FERREIRA; WEBER, 2015). The Oswaldo Cruz Foundation adds that the mission of the HMBs is to promote women's and children's health, by integrating and building partnerships with federal agencies, federal units, municipalities, the private sector and society, within the scope of the milk banks' activities (BRASIL, 2008).

The HMB plays an important role in caring for mothers and infants. To this end, it monitors premature and low birth weight infants, immunologically deficient infants, those with gastric disorders of various origins and those allergic to other types of milk. Also, mothers who have more breast milk than their child requires and who decide of their own free will to donate it, as well as women who are prevented from breastfeeding their children directly from the breast (VILLACA; FERREIRA;

WEBER, 2015; SILVA *et al.,* 2016).

■ Baby-Friendly Hospital Initiative

The BFHI was launched by the United Nations Children's Fund and the WHO, and aims to mobilize staff in units with obstetric services to change hospital practices and routines in order to promote, protect and support breastfeeding. To this end, the "ten steps to successful breastfeeding" have been established worldwide, with the fourth step dealing specifically with the importance of breastfeeding and skin-to-skin contact in the first few minutes of the baby's life (PEREIRA *et al.,* 2013; ESTEVES *et al.,* 2015).

The "ten steps" consist of a list of measures aimed at providing information to pregnant women and nursing mothers about the benefits and correct management of breastfeeding, offering materials that include guidelines for planning national programs, training for clinical teams and hospital managers, self-assessment forms and, finally, the accreditation of hospitals as "Friends of the Child" (PEREIRA *et al.,* 2013; LAMOUNIER, 2008).

The BFHI is a strategy based on the ability of NBs to interact with their mothers in the first few minutes of life, with the aim of increasing breastfeeding rates. The strategy of working with hospitals is due to the factors identified as unfavorable to breastfeeding, especially those related to misinformation and inadequate hospital routines (BEZERRA; TERRENGUI, 2011).

■ Joint Accommodation

Joint Lodging (JL) consists of a hospital principle in which the "healthy" NB, immediately after birth, remains at the mother's side 24 hours a day, in the same environment, until it is discharged from hospital. This system allows the puerperal woman to be encouraged to carry out all the care for the newborn. The CA aims to strengthen the emotional bonds between mother and baby from birth, to encourage early breastfeeding, and to provide emotional security for the parents in terms of caring for the baby (FARIA, 2010; BELO *et al.,* 2014).

The AC was created out of the need to provide better conditions for a good relationship between mother and child, from the very first minutes after giving birth, with the aim of promoting the indissolubility of the mother-child relationship, the humanization of care for hospitalized children, the possibility of shortening hospital stays, reducing the number of readmissions and the opportunity to provide health education (REIS *et al.,* 2008).

■ Amamenta Brasil and Alimenta Brasil Strategy

The Amamenta e Alimenta Brasil Strategy (EAAB) resulted from the integration of the actions of the Amamenta Brasil Network and the National Strategy for the Promotion of Healthy Complementary Feeding, and aims to promote reflection on the practice of health care for children aged 0 to 2 and the training of health professionals, through participatory activities, encouraging the exchange of experiences and the construction of knowledge based on local reality (MINISTÉRIO

DA SAÚDE, 2015).

The EAAB aims to qualify the work process of Primary Care (PC) professionals in order to reinforce and encourage the promotion of breastfeeding and healthy eating for children under two years of age within the scope of the Unified Health System (SUS). The Strategy also aims to reduce practices that discourage breastfeeding and complementary feeding in Basic Health Units (UBS), with the formation of healthy eating habits from infancy, an increase in the prevalence of children exclusively breastfed up to six months of age and complementary breastfeeding up to two years of age or more, as well as contributing to an improvement in the nutritional profile of children, with a reduction in nutritional deficiencies and excess or underweight (BRASIL, 2013).

3.3 Benefits of breastfeeding in the first hour of life

Breast milk contains all the nutrients needed by infants up to six months of age and is considered a key strategy for infant survival, due to its nutritional, immunological, economic-social and developmental benefits, which protect babies from common childhood diseases such as allergies and infections, important causes of infant morbidity and mortality, as well as its benefits for maternal health (ALMEIDA; LUZ; UED, 2014; ESTEVES *et al.*, 2015).

The advantages of breastfeeding are numerous and well known: with skin-to-skin contact shortly after birth, the newborn's intestine is colonized by microorganisms from the mother's skin flora. In addition, the transmission of heat from the mother's body to the NB keeps the baby warm, preventing hypothermia, and a sudden drop in temperature can lead to metabolic problems. This contact also helps to maintain acid-base balance, contributes to cardiorespiratory stability, favors the neonate's adaptation to extrauterine life and strengthens the affective bond between mother and child (MOREIRA *et al.*, 2014; SILVA *et al.*, 2016).

Pereira *et al* (2013) states that early skin-to-skin contact between mother and baby is also associated with better interaction between the two, longer total breastfeeding and the disappearance of the child's crying when in the mother's lap. In addition, there is an association between early breastfeeding and exclusive breastfeeding.

Early contact also provides the mother-baby binomial with the ability to love a human being, which happens right after birth, which is seen as a short period that brings long-term benefits. Valuing the first contact is of great importance to women, as it will remain with them for the rest of their lives (LEITE *et al.*, 2016). In addition, the act of breastfeeding is much more than simply the baby receiving milk from its mother, it is also a source of exchange of love and comfort, which are important for the child's psychological and emotional development (NUNES, 2015).

Early breastfeeding gives the newborn the chance to receive colostrum, which is highly nutritious, easily digestible and contains epidermal growth factor, which accelerates the maturation of the intestinal mucosa. It also contains bioactive immunological factors that protect the infant by preventing the intestinal colonization of pathogenic microorganisms. Colostrum juice also prevents the NB from physiological jaundice and hypoglycemia, which is often the reason for prescribing another type of milk as a food supplement for the child (MOURA *et al.*, 2014; ESTEVES *et al., 2014*).

The sucking of the nipple by the NB stimulates the maternal pituitary gland to produce prolactin and endogenous oxytocin, hormones that induce the production and ejection of milk, and which causes the uterus to contract and involute, preventing uterine atony, which is the primary cause of postpartum hemorrhage and, consequently, anemia (STRAPASSON, 2011; SÁ, 2015).

Breastfeeding soon after birth can prevent the introduction of drinks and/or food, which are a potential route for the entry of pathogens that cause damage to the newborn's intestine. It has also been identified as a protective factor for the use of artificial nipples (SÁ, 2015). The Ministry of Health states that breastfeeding provides families with a better quality of life, since children get sick less, and this reduces hospital visits and the use of medication to treat pathologies, which implies a good family relationship and, consequently, a reduction in costs (BRASIL, 2009).

3.4 Obstetric variables and breastfeeding in the first hour of life

Even though all the benefits of HFPA for mother and baby have been pointed out and proven, especially in terms of reducing neonatal morbidity and mortality, there are still many obstetric variables that prevent or delay the early start of breastfeeding. In 1989, the WHO and the United Nations Children's Fund (UNICEF) already pointed to the need to review the routines and procedures of health professionals and the organization of health services with the mother and child pair in labour and birth, since these could be acting as barriers to the start of breastfeeding, as well as its maintenance over time (SÁ, 2015).

With scientific progress and new discoveries in the field of asepsis, surgery, anesthesia, antibiotic therapy and hemotransfusion, hospital risks have decreased and interventions have increased, resulting in a progressive increase in caesarean sections. Hospital routines have also been created which, for supposedly scientific reasons or in order to better organize services, promote the separation of the mother from her newborn shortly after birth, with a negative impact on breastfeeding (STRAPASSON; FISCHER; BONILHA, 2011).

There are several "limiting" factors for APHV, such as HIV-positive mothers, as they are not advised to breastfeed their children due to the risk of vertical transmission of the disease through breast milk; low maternal schooling and low family income, as these mothers tend to start breastfeeding later, have greater difficulty understanding the importance of breastfeeding, and most of the time, access to health services for this population is more limited; maternal age of less than 25 years, as adolescent mothers are more likely not to start breastfeeding due to age-related insecurity and lack of self-confidence, fear of breastfeeding because they think it hurts, that the milk is insufficient and/or weak, among other myths (RODRIGUES *et al.*, 2013).

The absence of prenatal consultations and the lack of guidance on breastfeeding during prenatal care were also reported as factors associated with late initiation of breastfeeding. During prenatal care, mothers have the opportunity to receive information about pregnancy, breastfeeding and the health of mother and baby, as well as to prepare themselves to breastfeed "effectively" (SÁ, 2015; POSSOLLI *et al.*, 2015; BELO *et al.*, 2014).

Several studies have pointed to caesarean section as the main risk factor for non-APHV. Post-operative mothers find it more difficult to breastfeed, due to poor positioning and the mother's difficulty in touching the NB, since caesarean section delays or hinders the first feeds by altering the endocrine responses of the mother and the NB shortly after delivery, indicating that the surgical procedure causes pain and drowsiness, and the use of anaesthetics and analgesics affects the mother-baby interaction, which can cause disorganized behaviour in the baby and impair the spontaneous search for the breast of the nursing mother, as well as making it difficult for her to go to the AC (NARCHI, 2009; SILVA *et al.*, 2016).

Also cited as obstacles to the early start of breastfeeding were the policies and physical layout of institutions, which often do not guarantee privacy for women; the introduction of routines and procedures during labor and birth, most of which are unnecessary or could be carried out later; little encouragement from the health team for women to start breastfeeding; the administration of glucose water in bottles to newborns before the start of lactation; the early administration of milk formulas, among others (SÁ, 2015; SILVA *et al.*, 2016).

Individual factors, including advice and practices that weaken maternal confidence and self-efficacy, also negatively affect breastfeeding. Inadequate breastfeeding position or latch-on, the child's crying and fussing and the inability to calm the baby are common reasons for abandoning the practice. And the fact that mothers do not breastfeed successfully in their first pregnancy can interfere with breastfeeding in subsequent pregnancies (ROLINS *et al.*, 2016).

3.5 The role of nurses in promoting breastfeeding

Breastfeeding is not a simple process; it involves social, biological, psychological and cultural issues. Initially, the mother's wishes and decisions must be respected, but it is up to nurses to guide them in order to guarantee the best nutrition for the NB. Therefore, the clinical management of breastfeeding needs to be started during the NB, a period in which the woman already understands the physiology of lactation and the benefits for herself and the baby, allowing her to arrive at motherhood with this knowledge (ESTEVES *et al.*, 2015).

For early breastfeeding to be effective, mothers and babies need to have the support of all health professionals, especially nurses, from the time of PN, during delivery and in the postpartum period. Nurses are the professionals who are present throughout the pregnancy-puerperium cycle, and they must be able to conduct the PN and carry out nursing consultations, transmitting support and confidence, so that the pregnant woman can strengthen and lead the pregnancy, childbirth and decisions regarding the care of her child, including breastfeeding, with more autonomy

(STRAPASSON, 2011).

Nurses can be a determining factor in whether or not breastfeeding takes place, starting with their presence and posture at birth, providing early contact between mother and baby, stimulating APHV and offering support during the first feed. Nurses can work with other health professionals to inform them, raise their awareness and integrate them into programs to encourage, promote and support breastfeeding. To do this, they must seek scientific knowledge and develop technical and communication skills (STRAPASSON *et al.*, 2011; LEITE *et al.,* 2016).

It is therefore essential for the health team to play a welcoming role to mothers and babies, to always be available to listen and to clarify doubts and concerns, to encourage the exchange of experiences and, whenever necessary, to carry out a unique assessment of each case. The information and guidance provided should also be extended to the woman's family support network (ALMEIDA; LUZ; UED, 2014).

It is therefore important that all health professionals, especially nurses, develop competencies and skills in breastfeeding, with the aim of carrying out appropriate interventions and overcoming possible barriers to breastfeeding, especially in the delivery room, and better organizing and qualifying health services. It would also be essential to carry out pedagogical practices during the pregnancy-puerperium cycle, focusing on breastfeeding, with the main aim of preparing pregnant women to breastfeed their children and improving the quality of care for breastfeeding women and newborns.

Chapter 4

4 METHODS

This study is part of a research project developed by the Collective Health Research Group (GPESC), in the area of Child Health, entitled "Factors associated with breastfeeding in the first hour of life in children from Pico: a cross-sectional study".

4.1 Type of study

This is a descriptive, cross-sectional study with a quantitative approach. According to Gil (2010), the main objective of descriptive research is to describe the characteristics of a given population or phenomenon or to establish relationships between variables. One of its most significant characteristics is the use of standardized data collection techniques, such as the questionnaire.

Aragào (2011) says that cross-sectional studies visualize the situation of a population at a given time, as snapshots of reality. According to Dalfovo (2008), the quantitative method is characterized by the use of quantification, both in the way information is collected and in the way it is processed using statistical techniques, from the simplest to the most complex.

4.2 Place of study

The study was carried out in a public reference hospital in the municipality of Picos-PI.

Picos is a city in the southeastern region of Piauí, which is part of Macroregion 3 - Semiarid, the territory of the Guaribas Valley. Founded on December 12, 1890, it is at an altitude of 206m, 320km from Teresina (the state capital) and has an estimated population of 75,845 inhabitants in 2012 by the Brazilian Institute of Geography and Statistics (IBGE) (BRASIL, 2015).

According to the National Register of Health Establishments (CNES), the hospital currently has 133 beds, serves patients from 60 municipalities in the Picos macro-region, and has the following physical facilities: urgency and emergency with doctors' offices, minor surgery room, undifferentiated care room, plaster room, hygiene room, rest/observation room; outpatient with undifferentiated clinics, dentistry, outpatient surgery room, nursing room, immunization room, undifferentiated rest room and pediatric room; hospital with operating room, outpatient operating room, recovery room, normal delivery room, rooming-in beds, normal NB and pathological NB beds; support services with ambulance, sterilization center for materials, pharmacy, lactarium, laundry, morgue, Medical and Statistical Archive Service (SAME) or Patient Record Service (SPP), equipment maintenance service and social service (DATASUS, 2017).

4.3 Population and sample

The population consisted of all mothers whose children were born alive between January and December 2015. To estimate the size of the population, we used the number of mothers with live births at the hospital in 2013, totaling 924 mothers. The sample was census, as we worked with all the mothers of live births who met the eligibility criteria, totaling 587 mothers.

The participants were selected consecutively, as they were admitted to the hospital unit to give birth, and who met the eligibility criteria.

4.3.1 Exclusion criteria

- Mother of NB with very low birth weight, less than 1,500g or with gestational age (Capurro method) less than 32 weeks, which makes it impossible to stay in AC;
- Fetal or early neonatal death;
- Maternal death;
- Destination of the puerperal woman - semi-intensive care unit; and
- Mother with positive HIV serology in the PN recorded in medical records.

4.4 Study variables

In this study, 30 variables were studied, which will be mentioned below:

4.4.1 Socio-economic variables

- Maternal age: calculated in years;
- Schooling: calculated in years of study;
- Religion: computed as Catholic, Evangelical, Jehovah's Witness or No Religion;
- Family income: computed in minimum wages according to the salary in 2015;
- Maternal skin color: white, brown, black, yellow or indigenous;
- Marital status: married/stable union, single, divorced and widowed;
- Area of residence: was computed as rural or urban area; and
- Mother's occupation: she was counted as a farmer, housewife, unemployed, student, self-employed, among others.

4.4.2 Obstetric variables

- Did you have any PN consultations during the child's pregnancy: this was counted as yes or no;
- Number of NP consultations carried out: this was calculated in terms of the number of consultations registered and attended;
- Received guidance on breastfeeding in the PN: yes or no;
- Professionals who gave guidance on breastfeeding in the NP: nurse, doctor, nursing technician and Community Health Agent (CHA);
- Did you have any problems during pregnancy: yes or no;
- What problems were presented during pregnancy: bleeding, hypertensive syndrome, urinary infection, hypertension, threat of miscarriage, among others;
- Type of delivery: vaginal, caesarean or forceps;
- Problems during childbirth: yes or no;
- What problems were presented during childbirth: hypertension, dyspnea, hemorrhage, varicose veins, pre-eclampsia, among others;
- Did you have any problems after giving birth: yes or no;
- What problems did you have after giving birth: vomiting, headaches, bleeding, hypertension, nausea, etc;
- How long after giving birth did you breastfeed for the first time: it was calculated in minutes;
- Did you receive breastfeeding advice in hospital: yes or no;
- Breast problems: flat or inverted nipples, nipple cracks, breast engorgement, blocked ducts or mastitis and painful nipples;
- Breast examination: yes or no;
- Did you receive advice on how to treat breast problems: this was counted as yes, by the nurse; yes, by the nursing technician; yes, by the doctor; or no.

4.4.3 Biochemical variables

The data on these variables was taken from the pregnant woman's card.

- Has a blood test been carried out: yes or no;
- Tested for anemia: yes or no;
- Tested for syphilis: yes or no;
- Has a diabetes test been carried out: yes or no;
- HIV test: yes or no; and
- Has a urine test been carried out: yes or no.

4.5 Data collection

Data was collected between January and December 2015. A form adapted from other studies (BOCCOLINI *et al.*, 2011; CAMINHA et *al.,* 2010) was used to collect the data. The form contained information about the pregnancy and mother's PN, delivery conditions and APHV. The form was applied by trained nursing academics and was filled in with the mother in the shared accommodation of Ward A (Obstetrics) at the hospital.

4.6 Data analysis

Microsoft office Excel software version 2013 was used to build the database, and typing was standardized and carried out by a single person. Statistical Package for Social Sciences (SPSS) version 20.0 was used for statistical analysis. The data was organized in tables and graphs and analyzed using absolute and percentage frequencies, measures of central tendency and dispersion and association tests.

The Student's t-test for independent samples was used to compare means. To associate qualitative variables, Pearson's Chi-square test was used for expected frequencies greater than 5, and Fisher's and likelihood ratio tests for expected frequencies less than 5. To calculate the prevalence ratio of breastfeeding in the first hour of life, the Odds Ratio (OR) was calculated. For all the tests carried out, a p-value < 0.05 was considered.

4.7 Ethical aspects

To carry out the study, all the ethical principles contained in Resolution 466/2012 (BRASIL, 2013), which governs research involving human beings, were adopted. The research project was submitted to the Research Ethics Committee of the Federal University of Piauí and approved under opinion number 1.144.279 (ANNEX A).

The children's mothers and/or guardians were informed of the study's objectives and agreed to take part by signing the Informed Consent Form (ICF) (APPENDIX B) in two copies. For mothers under the age of 18, the consent of the legal guardian was requested, in which case the child's grandparents signed the ICF (APPENDIX C), in addition to the participating mother, who signed the Informed Consent Form (TALE) (APPENDIX D).

The risk of the study was that the "patient" would be embarrassed when answering the questions on the form, as it was completed in a collective room. The benefit of the study was greater knowledge of the factors that influence APHV in children in the municipality of Picos - PI.

Chapter 5

5 RESULTS

The following results deal with socioeconomic and demographic data, obstetric profile and data related to breastfeeding in the first hour of life.

Table 1 - Sociodemographic characteristics of the mothers surveyed. Picos, 2015. N = 587.

Variables	F	%
Age (in years)		
10-14	5	0,9
15-19	124	21,1
20-24	155	26,4
25-29	144	24,5
30-34	100	17,0
35-39	47	8,0
40 or more	4	0,7
Not informed	8	1,4
Education		
No schooling	5	0,9
Elementary school incomplete	59	10,1
Complete primary education	177	30,2

High school incomplete	84	14,3
Complete high school	144	24,5
Superior	78	13,3
Postgraduate studies	25	4,3
Not informed	15	2,4
Religion		
Catholic	458	78,0
Evangelical	82	14,0
Jehovah's Witness	6	1,0
No religion	33	5,6
Not informed	8	1,4
Family income (in minimum wages)		
<1	442	75,3
1 |- 2	87	14,8
2 |- 3	12	2,0
3 |- 4	4	0,7
4 or more	6	1,0
Not informed	36	6,2

Skin color		
White	134	22,8
Brown	376	64,1
Black	74	12,6
Yellow	2	0,3
Not informed	1	0,2
Marital Status		
Married/stable union	457	77,9
Single	113	19,3
Divorced	6	1,0
Not informed	11	1,8
Housing area		
Rural	318	54,2
Urban	255	43,4
You don't know	2	0,3
Not informed	12	2,1

Table 1 shows that the majority of the

Mothers (26.4%) were between 20 and 24 years old, and 30.2% had completed elementary school, with only 0.9% having no schooling.

With regard to type of religion, most of the mothers surveyed (78.0%) professed to be Catholic and 5.6% said they had no religion. With regard to family income, 75.3% reported having up to one minimum wage. The majority declared themselves to be brown (64.1%) and white (22.8%).

With regard to marital relations, 77.9% of the mothers reported being married or in a stable union with their partner and 19.3% were single during pregnancy. 54.2% reported living in rural areas.

Table 2 - Characterization of maternal occupation. Picos, 2015. N = 587.

Variables	F	%
Busy		
Farmer	179	35,0
Housewife	172	29,3
Unemployed	50	8,5
Student	41	7,0
Autonomous	19	3,2
Teacher	15	2,6
Domestic	13	2,2
General service	9	1,5
Saleswoman	9	1,5
Cashier operator	6	1,0
Diarist	5	0,8
Receptionist	5	0,9
Merchant	3	0,5

Nursing technician	3	0,5
ACS	3	0,5
Secretary	3	0,5
Seamstress	2	0,3
Businesswoman	2	0,3
Administrative assistant	2	0,3
Babysitting	1	0,2
Radio attendant	1	0,2
Gari	1	0,2
Credit and collection analyst	1	0,2
Dental assistant	1	0,2
Retired	1	0,2
Library assistant	1	0,2
Shop assistant	1	0,2
Caring for the elderly	1	0,2
Stockist	1	0,2
Director	1	0,2
Clerk	1	0,2

	N	%
Public servant	1	0,2
Store assistant	1	0,2
Nurse	1	0,2
Office assistant	1	0,2
Not informed	30	0,4

As shown in Table 2, the most prevalent maternal occupation among the mothers surveyed was: farmer/woman (35.0%), followed by housewife (29.3%) and unemployed (8.5%).

Table 3 - Distribution of mothers surveyed by prenatal data. Picos, 2015. N =587.

Variables	N	%
Prenatal Yes	573	97,6
No	12	2,0
Not informed	2	0,4
Number of PN consultations 1-5	115	19,6
6 or more	444	75,7
Not informed	28	4,7
Orientales on breastfeeding in the PN Yes	399	68,0
No	1/4	29,6
No PN	13	2,2

Variables	N	%
Not informed	1	0,2
Professional responsible for guidance Nurse	340	58,0
Medical	47	8,0
ACS	20	3,4
Doctor, Nurse and CHWs	3	0,4
Nursing technician	1	0,2
Did not receive guidance	175	29,8
You don't know	1	0,2
Problems during pregnancy Yes	110	18,7
No	469	79,9

	N	%
Not informed	8	1,4
Pregnancy problems (SIC')		
Bleeding	17	3,0
Hypertensive syndrome	17	3,0
Urinary infection	12	2,1
Hypertension	12	2,1

Amcaca dc aborto	9	1,5
Information	5	0,9
Hypotension	4	0,7
Dorcs	3	0,5
Syphilis	3	0,5
Alcrgia	2	0,3
Varizcs	2	0,3
Recalculation	2	0,3
Gcstational Diabctcs	2	0,3
Pre-eclampsia	2	0,3
Prccocc dilation	2	0,3
Kidney infection	2	0,3
Anemia	2	0,3
Fainting	1	0,2
Kidney enlargement	1	0,8
Ovarian cyst	1	0,2
Placental abruption	1	0,2
Electric shock	1	0,2
Car accident	1	0,2

Herniated disc	1	0,2
Thrombosis	1	0,2

According to the client

     According to Table 3, 97.6% of mothers had a prenatal visit, of which 75.7% had 6 or more visits. Of all the mothers, 68.0% received guidance on breastfeeding during prenatal care, 58% of which was offered by nurses, and 29.8% received no guidance at all.

Among the mothers surveyed, 18.7% reported having problems during pregnancy, the most common being hypertensive syndrome (3.0%), hemorrhage (3.0%), hypertension (2.1%), urinary infection (2.1%) and threatened abortion (1.5%).

Graph 1 - Characterization of the tests carried out during prenatal care. Picos, 2015. N = 587.

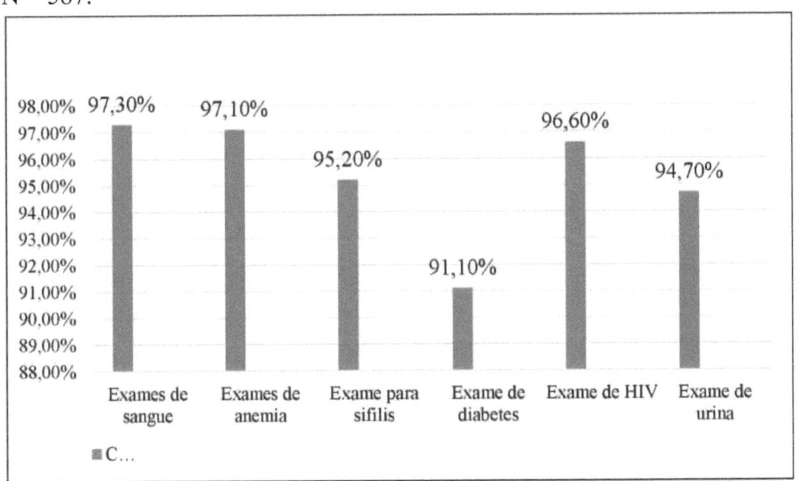

As shown in Graph 1, 97.3% of the mothers surveyed had undergone blood tests, 97.1% for anemia, 95.2% for syphilis, 91.1% for diabetes and 96.6% for HIV. With regard to urine testing, 94.7% reported having done so.

Table 4 - Obstetric characteristics of the mothers surveyed. Picos, 2015. N = 587.

Variables	F	%
Type of delivery Caesarean section	441	75,1
Vaginal	143	24,4

Forceps	2	0,3
Not informed	1	0,2
Problems during childbirth		
Yes	38	6,5
No	543	92,5
Not informed	2	1,0
Problems during childbirth (SIC')		
Hypertension	8	1,4
Dyspnea	7	1,2
Bleeding	3	0,5
Varicose veins	2	0,3
Pre-eclampsia	2	0,3
Hypotension	2	0,3
Bladder rupture	1	0,2
Loss of amniotic fluid	1	0,2
Changing the type of delivery	1	0,2

Circular cord	1	0,2
Muscle weakness	1	0,2
Problems after childbirth		
Yes	15	2,6
No	569	96,9
Not informed	3	0,5
Problems after giving birth (SIC')		
Vomit	5	0,9
Headache	2	0,3
Bleeding	1	0,2
Hypertension	1	0,2
Nausea	1	0,2
Bleeding	1	0,2

According to the client

According to table 4, the most prevalent type of delivery was caesarean section (75.1%). Of all the mothers, 6.5% had problems during childbirth, including hypertension (1.4%), dyspnea (1.2%), hemorrhage (0.5%), among others.

As for postpartum problems, only 2.6% of mothers had any, the most common being vomiting (0.9%) and headaches (0.3%).

Graph 2 - <u>Prevalence of breastfeeding in the first hour of life. Picos,</u> 2015. N=587

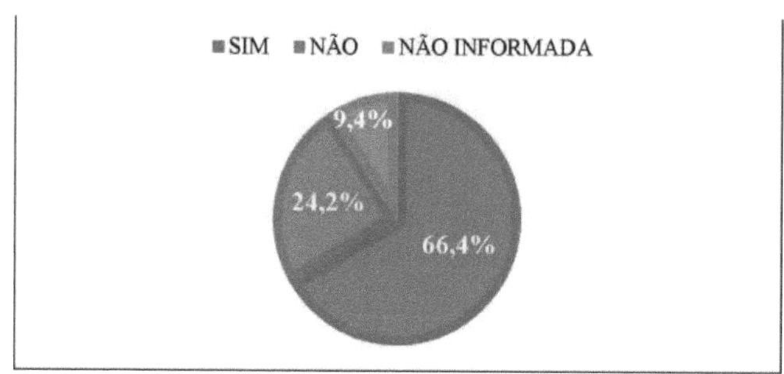

As can be seen in Graph 2, 66.4% of mothers breastfed their children within the first hour of birth.

Table 5 - Characterization of assistance to promote breastfeeding in the hospital unit. Picos, 2015. N = 587.

Variables	F	%
Guidance on breastfeeding in hospital		
Yes	160	27,3
No	424	72,2
Not informed	3	0,5
Breast examined		
Yes	224	38,2
No	347	59,1
Not informed	16	2,7
Breast problems		
None	525	89,4

Nipple fissure	20	3,4
Painful nipples	19	3,3
Flat or inverted nipples	13	2,2
Breast engorgement	4	0,6
Obstructed ducts and mastitis	3	0,5
Not informed	3	0,6
Guidance on treating breast problems		
No breast problems	502	85,5
No guidance	57	9,7
Yes, by the nurse	20	3,4
Yes, by the doctor	3	0,5
Yes, by the nursing technician	2	0,3
Not informed	3	0,6

Table 5 shows that 72.2% of mothers were not given breastfeeding advice in a hospital setting. Of the women studied, only 38.2% had their breasts examined.

With regard to breast problems, 3.4% of mothers reported having nipple cracks, 3.3% painful nipples, 2.2% flat or inverted nipples, among others. The professionals who gave advice on how to treat these problems were nurses (3.4%), doctors (0.5%) and nursing technicians (0.3%), while 9.7% of mothers did not receive any advice.

Table 6 - Relationship between socioeconomic variables and breastfeeding in the first hour of life. Picos, 2015. N = 587.

Socio-economic variables	Breastfeeding no the first hour		p-value	Rpa (95% CI)
	Yes	No		
Age¥	25,08 (6,20)	25,56 (6,37)	0,438€	-
Income¥	705,32 (1087,68)	749,74 (768,37)	0,667€	-
Skin color&			0,378£	-
White	86 (69,9)	37 (30,1)		
Brown	255 (75,7)	82 (24,3)		
Black	47 (68,1)	22 (31,9)		
Yellow	1 (50,0)	1 (50,0)		
Conjugal&			0,698£	-
Married	302 (72,2)	116 (27,8)		
Single	76 (76,0)	24 (24,0)		
Divorced	4 (80,0)	1 (20,0)		
Housing area&			0,006*	1,722 (1,163 - 2,550)
Rural	222 (78,2)	62 (21,8)		
Urban	158 (67,5)	76 (32,5)		

According to Table 6, breastfeeding was 70% higher among rural women compared to urban women. There was no statistically significant relationship between the other socio-economic variables and APHV among the children surveyed.

Table 7 - Association between "obstetric variables" and breastfeeding in the first hour of life. Picos, 2015. N = 587.

Obstetric variables	Breastfeeding in the first time		p-value	Rpa (95%CI)
	Yes	No		
Type of delivery			0,010£**	1,932 (1,162 -
Vaginal	103 (82,4%)	22 (17,6%)		3,210)
Caesarean section	286 (70,8%)	118 (29,2%)		
Prenatal care, in n (%)			0,303¥	-
Yes	380 (73,1)	140 (26,9)		
No	9 (90,0)	1 (10,0)		
Advised on breastfeeding in the PN in n (%)			0,216£	-
Yes	276 (75,0)	92 (25,0)		
No	106 (69,7)	46 (30,3)		

Problems during pregnancy, in n (%)			$0,400^{£}$	-
Yes	77 (77,0)	23 (23,0)		
No	309 (72,9)	115 (27,1)		
Problems during childbirth, in n (%)			$0,112^{£}$	-
Yes	23 (62,2)	14 (37,8)		
No	364 (74,1)	127 (25,9)		
Problems after childbirth, in n (%)			$1,000^{£}$	-
Yes	9 (75,0)	3 (25,0)		
No	380 (73,5)	137 (26,5)		

¥Fisher's exact test; £Pearson's chi-squared test; [a] Prevalence ratio; °Confidence interval.

The type of delivery showed a statistically significant relationship with breastfeeding. The occurrence of breastfeeding in the first hour of life was 90% higher among women who gave birth vaginally compared to those who had a caesarean section.

Chapter 6

6 DISCUSSION

This study analyzed the prevalence of breastfeeding in the first hour of life in children from Picos and investigated the risk factors related to early non-breastfeeding among mothers and NBs at a public reference hospital in the municipality of Picos-PI. To prepare the discussion, the results were analyzed and compared with the national and/or international scientific literature on the subject.

In the sample, the mothers had an average age of 22 years, with a range of 14 to 43 years. In a study conducted by Moura *et al* (2014), with 23 post-operative women in a maternity hospital in Minas Gerais, a similar average age was found, of 23 years, with a range of 21 to 25 years. A similar age was also identified in 40 pregnant women at a hospital in the northwest of Paraná, with a prevalence of ages between 21 and 29 (ANTUNES *et al.,* 2015).

In this study, there was no mean difference between the ages of women who breastfed or not in the first hour of life. However, according to Esteves *et al* (2014), younger women have a higher risk of delaying the early start of breastfeeding, and this finding may be related to their immaturity, greater inexperience and lack of preparation for motherhood. Other factors, such as the need to return to school, the existence or not of married life, as well as family influence in the face of the difficulties of breastfeeding, can influence the non-occurrence of breastfeeding and lead to early weaning (SOUTO, 2014).

When the level of maternal education was analyzed, most of the data showed that the women had only a few years of schooling. This result is in line with a study carried out in Minas Gerais, where almost all of the post-operative mothers in a maternity hospital had incomplete primary education (MOURA *et al.,* 2014). In a study carried out in Vitória - ES, most of the pregnant women (76.9%) in the sample had eight years or more of schooling (WILL *et al.,* 2013).

Low income prevailed in more than a third of the mothers studied. In a study carried out in Rio de Janeiro with the aim of analyzing the factors associated with the period between birth and the start of breastfeeding in mothers who underwent rapid HIV testing during hospitalization for childbirth, 28% of the mothers had an income of up to one minimum wage (POSSOLLI *et al.,* 2015).

According to Moura *et al* (2014), mothers with low levels of schooling and low income deserve special attention from the Family Health Strategy (ESF), as well as from professionals working in hospital settings, since a lack of basic school knowledge makes it difficult to understand the benefits and practice of breastfeeding, as well as negatively interfering in the development of mothers' commitment to breastfeeding, and is associated with an early return to labor (ANTUNES *et al.,* 2015; BROD; ROCHA; SANTOS, 2016).

With regard to the skin color of the participants, just over half of them declared themselves to be brown. A study carried out with the aim of verifying the factors that interfere with APHV in 403 puerperal women at a maternity hospital in Rio de Janeiro found lower values than these, where 45% of the women were brown (PEREIRA *et al.*, 2013). In a hospital in Recife - PE, a prevalence of 71.4% of brown women was found among AC mothers (BELO *et al.*, 2014).

In this study, skin color did not affect the outcome of breastfeeding. However, in a study carried out in Rio de Janeiro, women who reported their skin color as non-black were protected from APHV. From an economic and social point of view, black women are more susceptible to not breastfeeding early, since they have a lower level of education, are poor, and live in places with poor basic sanitation coverage, where access to prenatal consultations is also more limited (PEREIRA *et al.*, 2013).

Most of the women in the study were married/stable at the time of pregnancy/childbirth. Antunes *et al* (2015) found a similar result in a study carried out in a hospital in Paraná, in which 77.5% of the mothers were living with a partner at the time of the study. An even higher prevalence was found in a maternity hospital in Minas Gerais, where 91.3% of the puerperal women taking part in the study were married/stable partners (MOURA *et al.,* 2014).

In this study, the fact that the mothers were married or not did not have any influence on early breastfeeding, but Rodrigues *et al* (2013) states that the fact that the mother receives support from her husband/partner during the pregnancy-puerperal period has a positive influence on the early initiation and maintenance of breastfeeding.

More than two-thirds of the mothers in the study had some kind of occupation/work during pregnancy/childbirth. A lower result was found in a study conducted by Antunes *et al* (2015), in which 65% of the mothers who were treated at a hospital in Paraná had a job. In a maternity hospital in Rio de Janeiro, 51.9% of women worked outside the home (PEREIRA *et al.*, 2013).

Among the professions found in this study, the most prevalent were farmers (35%) and housewives (29.3%), and less than a tenth of the mothers were unemployed. A study of pregnant women in a municipality in Vitória, Espírito Santo, found a similar maternal occupation, where 44.4% of the women were housewives and only 2.6% were unemployed (WILL *et al.*, 2013).

Maternal work has been cited by some authors as a factor that has negative effects on breastfeeding. Mothers who work outside the home are a potential risk group for not starting breastfeeding or for early weaning. Short maternity leave leads to a fourfold increase in the chance of not starting breastfeeding. This group of women requires special attention from health professionals, who plan specific strategies to protect the initiation and continuity of breastfeeding for children, through individualized and systematized support for the mother-child dyad (OLIVEIRA *et al.*, 2014; ROLINS *et al.*, 2016).

The prevalence of breastfeeding in the first hour of life in this survey was almost two-thirds of mothers. Data from the 2nd Breastfeeding Prevalence Survey in the Capitals and Federal District revealed that 67.7% of Brazilian children were breastfed in the first hour of life (BRASIL, 2009). Consistent results were found in a study carried out by Antunes *et al* (2015) with 40 pregnant women in a hospital in Paraná, in which APHV had a frequency of 63%. A survey of 191 women from an

Islampur village in Upramilla of Dhamrai under Dhaka District showed a prevalence of early breastfeeding of 56.54% (RAHMAN *et al.*, 2014).

A study aimed at verifying the factors that interfere with APHV among 403 puerperal women in a maternity hospital in Rio de Janeiro found a lower result, with a prevalence of 43.9%, 27.9% of children born by caesarean section and 52.5% of those born by vaginal delivery having been breastfed within the first hour of life (PEREIRA *et al.*, 2013).

These results show us the importance of investing in the implementation of the fourth step of the BFHI in all hospitals/maternities, since early contact should be encouraged with all clinically stable NBs whose mothers are able to breastfeed, taking advantage of the fact that in the first hour of life, the baby remains alert and can easily find the nipple and start breastfeeding (LEITE *et al.*, 2016; MOURA et al., 2014; ANTUNES *et al.,* 2015).

For mother and NB to enjoy the greatest benefits from breastfeeding, it should be started as early as possible, as breastfeeding from the first day of life can prevent 16% of neonatal deaths. This rate can rise to 22% if breastfeeding is brought forward to the first hour after birth, representing a considerable increase in reducing the risk of death at a crucial stage for the child's survival and development (BELO *et al.*, 2014).

Boccolini *et al* (2013) observed in a study conducted in Brazil with more than 10,000 children that APHV is essentially determined by the maternity hospital where the birth takes place, and that individual factors such as age, parity and maternal education do not play a significant role. She also says that mothers' feelings and wishes are not always respected during childbirth, and that in this moment of fragility, professional conduct can be a determining factor in breastfeeding in the delivery room. Sá (2015) also states that mothers have little or no decision-making power over the early breastfeeding of their children, being limited to the practices of the professionals involved in childbirth and the institutional routines in force in maternity hospitals.

In this study, caesarean section was the risk factor most strongly associated with late initiation of breastfeeding. This type of delivery was more than two-thirds prevalent among the mothers in the study, five times higher than what is considered acceptable by the WHO (10 to 15%), and was almost double that of a study carried out with women from a hospital in Recife (40%) (BELO *et al.*, 2014). In a review of the literature, which aimed to verify the factors associated with non-APHV, the proportion of caesarean sections ranged from 2.1% in a survey in rural Ethiopia to 49.3% in a hospital sample in the city of Rio de Janeiro (ESTEVES *et al.,* 2014).

This mode of delivery has been described as an important barrier to the timely initiation of breastfeeding, generally due to post-operative care routines that delay or interrupt contact between mother and child in the postpartum period (ESTEVES *et al.*, 2014; ESTEVES *et al.,* 2015). Behavioral factors are also involved in this relationship, so that mothers undergoing caesarean sections would be less inclined to breastfeed (CARVALHO *et al.*, 2016). Although caesarean sections increase the risk of maternal death, puerperal infections and can reduce the prevalence of APHV by half, the proportion of deliveries by this route has increased and is a cause for concern worldwide (MOURA *et al.*, 2014).

The proportion of vaginal deliveries occurred in less than a quarter of the mothers studied. Antunes *et al* (2015) found an even lower result, 17.5% of vaginal deliveries in a hospital in the northwestern region of Paraná, and of these, only 5% breastfed within the first hour of life. However, in a study carried out in a hospital in Rio de Janeiro, which aimed to verify the factors associated with late breastfeeding, a prevalence of 67.8% of vaginal deliveries was found (ESTEVES *et al.*, 2015).

According to our study, the occurrence of breastfeeding in the first hour of life was 90% higher among women who gave birth vaginally compared to those who had a caesarean section. A higher result was found in a national survey carried out by Carvalho *et al* (2016), in which mothers who had a vaginal delivery were 98% more likely to breastfeed in the first hour of life compared to those who had a caesarean section.

Vaginal delivery was considered to be protective against APHV. Authors state that women who give birth vaginally have a more active participation during and after delivery; they go to the room/shared accommodation in a shorter time, when compared to cases of caesarean section; and there are greater possibilities for the baby to be placed naked in direct contact with their body in the first few minutes after birth, allowing the mother to identify signs in the child that they are ready to breastfeed (PEREIRA *et al.*, 2013; ANTUNES *et al.*, 2015).

When analyzing the living areas of the women under study, it became clear that just over half of them lived in rural areas, and that less than half lived in urban areas. Studies carried out in Brazilian states such as Bahia (DEMÉTRIO; PINTO; ASSIS, 2012) and Piauí (RAMOS *et al.*, 2008) showed somewhat similar results, with 29.8% of the women living in urban areas and 70.2% in rural areas, and 85.3% living in rural areas and 14.7% in urban areas, respectively.

The fact that mothers lived in urban areas was the second factor identified as a risk factor for not breastfeeding early. Living in a rural area was the second protective factor for the outcome of breastfeeding in the first hour. The fact that women lived in rural areas increased the chances of their newborn being breastfed in the first hour of life by 70% when compared to those who lived in urban areas.

Contradictory results were found in a systematic literature review carried out by Esteves *et al* (2014), which showed that living in a rural area was a risk factor in two studies carried out in African countries and a protective factor in two Asian studies. In a study carried out in the state of Piauí, the fact that mothers lived in rural areas increased the percentage of breastfeeding by 88% when compared to urban dwellers (RAMOS *et al.*, 2008). In a study carried out in Rio de Janeiro, the area of residence was not associated with the outcome of breastfeeding (POSSOLLI *et al.*, 2015).

The literature does not clearly show why rural areas are protective of early breastfeeding, but according to Demétrio, Pinto and Assis (2012), living in rural areas entails a lower risk of early interruption of exclusive and total breastfeeding, since fewer women work outside the home and they are less influenced by advertisements for breastmilk substitutes when compared to mothers in urban areas.

This study found that almost all of the mothers underwent prenatal care, with more than a third of them having six or more appointments and more than half of these women receiving guidance on breastfeeding during these meetings. These findings are consistent, to a certain extent, with a study of 573 mothers from a hospital in Recife, which showed that 98% of women received prenatal care, 55.2% of these women received guidance during prenatal care on the importance of breastfeeding and 72.1% received six or more consultations (BELO *et al.*, 2014).

Pereira *et al* (2013) also found a similar result in a study of 403 puerperal women in a maternity hospital in Rio de Janeiro, in which 93.1% of the mothers had prenatal care, 55.6% had received information about breastfeeding during this period and 56.6% had 6 to 12 consultations. These data also corroborate the findings of a study carried out with 191 women from an Islampur village in Dhaka, where 84.3% received prenatal care and of these, 84.47% received guidance on breastfeeding (RAHMAN *et al.*, 2014).

This study showed no relationship between APHV, prenatal care and receiving breastfeeding advice during the PN. However, contradictory literature has been found. A study carried out in a maternity hospital in Rio de Janeiro showed that the mothers interviewed who had undergone prenatal care were strongly protected in terms of breastfeeding their children in the first hour of life (PEREIRA *et al.*, 2013). Moura *et al* (2014), reported an association between APHV and having received guidance on the advantages of breastfeeding in the PN, indicating that this support favors preparation for breastfeeding, and that women who did not receive guidance on breastfeeding before giving birth had more difficulty maintaining breastfeeding.

During prenatal care, women have a great opportunity to receive important information that can be decisive for breastfeeding. It is therefore necessary for mothers to carry out this follow-up in accordance with the recommendations of the Prenatal and Birth Humanization Program (PHPN), which states that all pregnant women should have at least six consultations, as this is the minimum follow-up to be carried out in order to increase subsidies to reduce maternal and perinatal mortality and neonatal morbidity and mortality (BROD; ROCHA; SANTOS, 2016).

Prenatal care should reflect comprehensive care (care, prevention and health promotion). Studies show that different indicators of access (number of consultations) and quality (iron prescription, breastfeeding guidance, home visits) of prenatal care have been identified as factors associated with the timely initiation of breastfeeding. The information that health professionals give pregnant women during consultations favors preparation for breastfeeding and can contribute to breastfeeding while still in the delivery room (ESTEVES *et al.*, 2014).

With regard to the guidance and information on breastfeeding received in the hospital setting, the municipality of Picos was "poorly" supported by health professionals in this phase of care, since less than a third of mothers received support and guidance on establishing and maintaining breastfeeding.

A study carried out in the United Kingdom with mothers of full-term and late preterm newborns found that when breastfeeding guidance was given in hospital, through support groups, there was a greater likelihood of breastfeeding occurring over a shorter period of time. The author also states that mothers who reported having received little help were less likely to maintain breastfeeding for a longer period of time (OLIVEIRA *et al.*, 2015).

The influence of guidance and support in this scenario, where the mother has her first encounter with breastfeeding, is notorious, and professionals need to be prepared to guide and encourage this practice (LIMA; SOUZA, 2013; ESTEVES *et al.*, 2014). Prates *et al* (2014) adds that during this assistance, attention should also be paid to the socio-historical-cultural factors that can directly influence the act of breastfeeding.

It is known that the practice of breastfeeding is very important, and in addition to willpower, it is necessary for mothers to be aware of the breast problems that can occur, how to identify them and, above all, how to prevent them, as they are among the main factors that lead to early weaning (BRASIL, 2009). In addition, it is of the utmost importance that health professionals pay attention to examining women's breasts in order to identify possible "inconveniences" that could delay the start of breastfeeding.

When analyzing the frequency of breast complications associated with breastfeeding, it can be seen that a small proportion of mothers had some kind of breast problem, the most prevalent being nipple cracks, painful nipples and flat or inverted nipples. A study conducted by Rahman *et al* (2014) in Dhamrai (Dhaka District) found similar breast problems to those found in this study, where 25.72% of the mothers had cracked nipples, 11.43% had inverted nipples and 5.72% had mastitis. In Mato Grosso, a study aimed at verifying the relationship between breastfeeding and the complications that contribute to early weaning also frequently found difficulties in the lactation process, such as inverted or flat nipples and nipple cracks (OLIVEIRA *et al.*, 2015).

In this study, just over a third of women had their breasts examined by a health professional during the pregnancy-puerperium process. Almost double this result was found in a hospital in Recife, where 66.4% of women had their breasts assessed during the PN (BELO *et al.*, 2014)

It is known that vulnerability to breast complications can be significantly reduced through prophylactic and curative interventions. This requires effective guidance on positioning, correct latch-on and manual milking, from the first breastfeeding, through the hospitalization period, to puerperium consultations. Sunbathing is recommended to prevent fissures, as it keeps the nipples dry and prevents skin maceration (LIMA; SOUSA, 2013).

With regard to the blood tests requested during prenatal consultations, almost all the mothers had them done. And when it came to the HIV test, 96.6% of the women had it while still in the prenatal period. A study carried out in hospitals in Rio de Janeiro found lower rates of HIV testing, where 79% of mothers reported having undergone HIV testing during prenatal care (POSSOLLI *et al.*, 2015).

Not knowing one's HIV status was identified by Esteves *et al* (2015) as an independent risk factor for late initiation of breastfeeding. HIV testing in the PN and maternity ward is essential for preventing vertical transmission of the virus. Although our country has a program of well-established protocols for the prevention and control of HIV/AIDS, flaws are still found in the processes involved.

In this study, very few women had health problems during prenatal/partum/postpartum care, with the highest prevalence being bleeding, hypertension and vomiting, respectively. The fact that women had any complications showed no significant relationship with the early start of breastfeeding. However, a study carried out in Recife showed that among maternal factors, severe pre-eclampsia was the main limitation for not starting APHV. In addition, hypertensive disorders during pregnancy substantially increase morbidity in newborns, with the need for special care (BELO *et al.*, 2014).

Breastfeeding in the first hour of life is therefore considered a key strategy for promoting and protecting health, given its numerous benefits for the mother-child binomial. It should be encouraged and implemented as a hospital routine in all countries, with the aim of reducing maternal and neonatal morbidity and mortality. To this end, policies to promote breastfeeding that are appropriate to each context should be developed, with the aim of encouraging health professionals to be more holistic and to carry out interventions according to the particularities of each situation.

CONCLUSION

This study, designed to analyze the influence of obstetric variables on breastfeeding in the first hour of life at the public referral hospital in Picos, PI, showed that just over half of the women who gave birth in 2015 started breastfeeding in the first hour of life. This proportion was significantly higher among mothers who gave birth vaginally and who lived in rural areas. Caesarean section and the fact that the mothers lived in the urban area were the conditions identified as risk factors for late initiation of breastfeeding.

The main difficulties in carrying out this study were the mothers' refusal to take part in the research; their fear of providing certain information, especially in relation to monthly family income; and the students' lack of availability and/or commitment to collect the data in the morning, before the women were discharged from hospital. Another factor that influenced the collection was the fact that the information depended on the mothers' memory bias, as they were asked for the information, and sometimes they didn't remember certain pieces of information.

The results of this study suggest that factors related to childbirth care have the greatest influence on the timely initiation of breastfeeding. Even though we know that the continuity of breastfeeding depends on a complex network of social and cultural determinants, the timely start of breastfeeding is influenced by the hospital practices established by the institution. Health professionals, especially nurses, therefore have a responsibility and commitment to promote timely breastfeeding and good care practices for women and newborns.

It is therefore important to have scientific knowledge, technical skills and personal involvement in order to improve work processes with positive results. Continuing education for all health professionals is also necessary, as they take on the role of standardizing and regulating breastfeeding, based on constructed scientific knowledge, and must act with ethics and respect, in a scenario where health promotion and the reduction of morbidity and mortality must be considered priorities when defining public policies aimed at women's and children's health.

In view of the above, it is hoped that the results of this study will contribute to understanding the factors that influence breastfeeding in the first hour of life in the city surveyed. And so it can raise awareness among managers and health professionals to develop more effective educational and control measures, resulting in campaigns aimed at raising awareness in a more effective, humanizing way and, above all, so that mothers can see breastfeeding as much more than just a token of love, but as the best choice for feeding their children.

REFERENCES

ADUGNA, D. T. *et al.* Women's perception and risk factors for delayed initiation of breastfeeding in Arba Minch Zuria, Southern Ethiopia. **Int. Breastfeed J.,** v. 9, n. 8, p. 435-442, 2014.

AGUAYO, M. J. ROMERO, E. D. HERNANDEZ, A. M. T. Influencia de la atención al parto y al nacimiento sobre la lactancia, com especial atención a las cesáreas. **Evid. Pediatr.,** v. 7, n. 2, p. 102-110, 2011.

ALMEIDA, J. M.; LUZ, S. A. B.; UED, F. V. Support for breastfeeding by health professionals: an integrative literature review. **Rev. Paul. Pediatr.,** v. 33, n. 3, p. 355-362, 2014.

ANTUNES, M. B. *et al.* Factors associated with impediments to early breastfeeding: a descriptive study. **Braz. J. Nurs.,** v. 14, n.1, p. 525-533, 2015.

ARAGÁO, J. Introduction to quantitative studies used in scientific research. **Revista Práxis,** v.8, n.6, p.59-62, 2011.

AZEVEDO, A. R. M. *et al.* The clinical management of breastfeeding: nurses' knowledge. **Esc. Anna Nery,** v. 19, n. 3, p. 339-345, 2015.

BELO, M. N. M. *et al.* Breastfeeding in the first hour of life in a child-friendly hospital: prevalence, associated factors and reasons for non-occurrence. **Rev. Bras. Saúde Matern. Infant.,** v. 14, n. 1, p. 65-72, 2014.

BEZERRA, J. F.; TERRENGUI, L. C. S. Evaluation of the promotion, protection and support of breastfeeding. **Rev. Enferm. UNISA,** v.12, n.1, p.5-11, 2011.

BOCOLINI, C. S. *et al.* Breastfeeding in the first hour of life and neonatal mortality. **J. Pediatr.,** v. 89, n. 2, p. 131-136, 2013.

BOCOLINI, C. S. *et al.* Breastfeeding in the first hour of life and neonatal mortality. **Rev. Soc. Bol. Ped.** v. 54, n. 3, p. 141-47, 2015.

BORGES, J. H. **Breastfeeding in the first hour of life**. 2011. 21 f. Monograph (Graduation course in nursing) - Department of Life Sciences, Universidade Regional do Noroeste do Estado do Rio Grande do Sul, Ijuí, 2011.

BRAZIL. National Health Surveillance Agency. **Human milk bank**: operation, prevention and risk control / National Health Surveillance Agency. Brasília: Anvisa, 2008.

. Ministry of Health. National Health Council. **Resolution 466/12**. Brasília, 2013.

. Ministry of Health. **Ten steps to healthy eating**. 2. ed. Brasília: Série A. Normas e Manuais Técnicos, 2010.

. Ministry of Health. **National strategy to promote breastfeeding and healthy complementary feeding in the single health system**. Brasília, 2015a.

. Ministry of Health. **II Pesquisa de Prevalência de Aleitamento Materno nas Capitais Brasileiras e Distrito Federal**. Brasília: Ministry of Health Publishing House; 2009.

. Ministry of Health. Ministry of Planning, Planning and Management. Brazilian Institute of Geography and Statistics. **Intercensal interpolation and projections**. Rio de Janeiro: IBGE, 2015.

. Ministry of Health. Children's health. **Infant nutrition**: breastfeeding and complementary feeding. Brasilia, 2009a.

BROD, F. R.; ROCHA, D. L. B.; SANTOS, R. P. Knowledge and practices of mothers of premature newborns in the mainteining of breastfeeding. **J. Res. Fundam. Care**, v. 8, n. 4, p. 5108-5113, 2016.

BUENO, K. C. V. N. **The importance of exclusive breastfeeding up to six months of age for the promotion of health for mother and baby**. 2013. 28 f. Monograph (Specialized in Primary Care in Family Health) - Federal University of Minas Gerais, Campos Gerais, 2013.

CAMINHA, M. F. C. *et al.* Historical, scientific, socioeconomic and institutional aspects of breastfeeding. **Rev. Bras. Saúde Matern. Infant.**, v.10, n.1, p. 25-37, 2010.

CAMINHA, M. F. C. *et al.* Temporal trends and factors associated with the duration of breastfeeding in Pernambuco. **Rev. Saúde Pública.** v.2, n.44, p.240-248, 2010.

CARVALHO, K. E. G. *et al.* History and memories of the human milk bank of the Instituto de Medicina Integral Prof. Fernando Figueira (1987-2009) in Recife, Pernambuco, Brazil. **Rev. Bras. Saúde Matern. Infant.**, Recife, v. 10, n. 4, p. 477481, 2010.

CARVALHO, M. L. *et al.* The baby-friendly hospital initiative and breastfeeding at birth in Brazil: a cross sectional study. **Reproductive Health**, v. 13, n. 3, p. 207-215, 2016.

CASTRO, K. F. *et al.* Breast complications related to lactation. **O mundo da saúde,** v. 33, n.4, p. 433-39, 2009.

CERQUEIRA, P. A. **Factors associated with exclusive breastfeeding in the first month of age**. 2015. 69 f Dissertation (Master's Degree in Collective Health) - Postgraduate Program in Collective Health, State University of Feira de Santana, Feira de Santana, 2015.

NATIONAL COUNCIL OF HEALTH SECRETARIES. **Technical note 23/2013**. Brasilia, 2013.

DALFOVO, M. S.; LANA, R. A.; SILVEIRA, A. Métodos quantitativos e qualitativos: um resgate teórico. **Revista Interdisciplinar Científica Aplicada**, v.2, n.4, p.01- 13, 2008.

DEMÉTRIO, F.; PINTO, E. J.; ASSIS, A. M. O. Factors associated with early interruption of breastfeeding: a birth cohort study in two municipalities of Recôncavo da Bahia, Brazil. **Cad. Saúde Pública**, v. 28, n. 4, p. 641654, 2012.

ESTEVES, T. M. B. *et al.* Factors associated with breastfeeding in the first hour of life: a systematic review. **Rev. Saúde Pública,** v. 48, n. 4, p. 697-703, 2014.

ESTEVES, T. M. B. *et al.* Factors associated with late initiation of breastfeeding in hospitals of the Unified Health System in the city of Rio de Janeiro, Brazil, 2009. **Cad. Saúde Pública,** v. 31, n. 11, p. 2390-2400, 2015.

FARIA, A. C.; MAGALHÂES, L.; ZERBETTO, S. R. Implementation of rooming-in: difficulties faced in the perception of a nursing team. **Rev. Eletr. Enf.,** v. 12, n. 4, p. 669-677, 2010.

GIL, A. C. **Como elaborar projetos de pesquisa**. 5. ed. Sâo Paulo: Atlas, 2010.

GRANJA, D. M. A.; CUNHA, M. C. Breastfeeding and artificial breastfeeding throughout history: socio-cultural aspects. **Disturb. Comum,** v. 23, n. 2, p. 237-238, 2011.

LAMOUNIER, J. A. *et al.* Iniciativa Hospital Amigo da Crianza, mais de uma década no Brasil: repensando o futuro. **Rev. Paul. Pediatr.,** v. 26, n. 2, p. 161-169, 2008.

LEITE, M. F. F. S. *et al.* Promotion of breastfeeding in the first hour of the newborn's life by nursing professionals. **Arq. Cienc. Saúde UNIPAR,** v. 20, n. 2, p, 137-143, 2016.

LIMA, L. S. SOUZA, L. N. D. H. Maternal perception of the support received for breastfeeding: from the perspective of programmatic vulnerability. **Semina: Ciencias Biológicas e da Saúde,** v. 34, n. 1, p. 73-90, 2013.

MARQUES, A. N. **What the literature says about skin-to-skin contact between mother and newborn during caesarean section**: in search of arguments for good practices in birth care. 2016. 45 f. Monograph (Specialization in Obstetric Nursing) - School of Nursing, Federal University of Rio Grande do Sul and Federal University of Minas Gerais, Porto Alegre, 2016.

MONTEIRO, J. C. S.; NAKANO, A. M. S.; GOMES, F. A. Breastfeeding as a constructed practice. Reflections on the historical evolution of breastfeeding and early weaning in Brazil. **Invest. Educ. Enferm.,** v. 29, n.2, p. 315-321, 2011.

MOREIRA M. E. L. *et al.* Hospital care practices for healthy newborns in Brazil. **Cad. Saúde Pública,** v. 8, n. 3, p. 128-139, 2014.

MOURA, K. C. C. *et al.* Perceptions of puerperal women about the benefits of breastfeeding in the first hour of life. **Cogitare Enferm.,** v. 19, n. 1, p. 123-128, 2014.

NARCHI, N. Z. *et al.* Variables that influence the maintenance of exclusive breastfeeding. **Rev. Esc. Enferm. USP,** v. 43, n. 1, p.87-94, 2009.

NUNES, L. M. Importance of breastfeeding today. **Boletim Científico de Pediatria,** v. 4, n. 3, p. 55-58, 2015.

ODDY, W. H. Breastfeeding in the first hour of life protects against neonatal mortality. **J. Pediatr.**, v.89, n.2, p.109-111, 2013.

OLIVEIRA, C. N. T.; OLIVEIRA, M. V. Prevalence of exclusive breastfeeding and factors associated with early weaning in the municipality of Vitória da Conquista - BA. **Revista Eletrônica da Fainor**, v.5, n.1, p.160-174, 2012.

OLIVEIRA, C. S. *et al.* Breastfeeding and the complications that contribute to early weaning. **Rev. Gaúcha Enferm.**, v. 36, n. 4, p. 16-23, 2015.

PEREIRA, C. R. V. S. *et al.* Evaluation of factors that interfere with breastfeeding in the first hour of life. **Rev. Bras. Epidemiol**, v. 16. n. 2, p. 525-534, 2013.

POSSOLLI, G. T.; CARVALHO, M. L.; OLIVEIRA, M. I. C. Maternal HIV testing and initiation of breastfeeding: a survival analysis. **Jornal de Pediatria**, v. 91, n. 4, p. 397-404, 2015.

PRATES, L. A.; SCHMALFUSS, J. M.; LIPINSKI, J. M. Breastfeeding: family influence and the role of health professionals. **Rev. Enferm. UFSM**, v.4, n.2, p.359367, 2014.

RAGHAVAN, V. *et al.* First hour initiation of breastfeeding and exclusive breastfeeding at six weeks: prevalence and predictors in a tertiary care setting. **The Indian Journal of** Pediatrics, v. 81, n. 8, p. 743 - 750, 2014.

RAHMAN, M. *et al.* Breast Feeding Practices among Rural Women in a selected area of Bangladesh. **Northern International Medical College Journal**, v. 5, n. 2, 2014.

RAMOS, C. V. *et al.* Diagnosis of the breastfeeding situation in Piauí, Brazil. **Cad. Saúde Pública**, v.24, n.8, p.1753-1762, 2008.

REIS, K. S. *et al.* Programs to encourage breastfeeding. **Revista Digital de Nutrição**, v. 2, n. 3, p. 1-13, 2008.

ROCHA, S. The benefits of breast milk. **Rev. Eletr. Enf.**, v.15, n.1, p.253-264, 2013.

RODRIGUES, A. P. *et al.* Breastfeeding maintenance in preterm newborns: an integrative literature review. **Rev. Eletr. Enf.**, v.15, n.1, p.253-264, 2013.

ROLINS, N. C. *et al.* Why invest and what it will take to improve breastfeeding practices. **The Lancet**, v. 387, n. 1, p. 25-44, 2016.

SÁ, N. N. B. *et al.* Factors linked to health services determine breastfeeding in the first hour of life in the Federal District, Brazil, 2011. **Rev. Bras. Epidemiol**, v. 19, n. 3, p. 509-524, 2016.

SÁ, N. N. B. **Factors associated with breastfeeding in the first hour of life.** 2015. Thesis (Health Sciences) - Faculty of Health Sciences, University of Brasília, Brasília, 2015.

SILVA, C. M. *et al.* Factors associated with skin-to-skin contact between mother and child and breastfeeding in the delivery room. **Rev. Nutr.**, v. 29, n. 4, p. 457-471, 2016.

SOUTO, D. C.; JAGER, M. E.; DIAS, A. C. G. Breastfeeding and the occurrence of early weaning in adolescent puerperal women. **Revista de**

Atençâo à Saúde, v. 12, n. 41, p.73-79, 2014.

SOUZA, A. B. G. **Enfermagem neonatal: cuidado integral ao recém-nascido.** 1. ed. Sâo Paulo: Martinari, 2011.

STRAPASSON, M. R. *et al.* Breastfeeding in the first hour of life in a private hospital in Porto Alegre/RS - experience report. **R. Enferm.**, v.1, n.3, p.489- 496, 2011.

UNICEF. **World situation of children**: 2013. Children with disabilities. Brasilia: UNICEF; 2013. [accessed on Nov. 11, 2013]. Available at: http://www.unicef.org/brazil/pt/PT_SOWC2013.pdf.

VILLAÇA, L. M. S.; FERREIRA, A. G. S.; WEBER, L. C. The importance of breastfeeding for the mother-child binomial made available by the human milk bank. **Rev. Saúde AJES**, v. 1, n. 2, p. 1-19, 2015.

WILHELM, L. A. *et al.* The experience of breastfeeding from the perspective of women: contributions for nursing. **Rev. Enferm. UFSM**, v.5, n.1, p.160-168, 2015.

WILL, T. K. *et al.* Protective factors for breastfeeding in the first hour of life. **Rev. Bras. Promoc. Saude**, v.26, n.2, p.274-280, 2013.

APPENDICES
APPENDIX A - Data collection form

ORDER No. (crianza)   DATE OF COLLECTION:

____ // ___

FAMILY INCOME:reaisRELIGION   :
MOTHER'S SCHOOLING: years of study MOTHER'S AGE:
years MATERNAL OCCUPATION:

DATA COLLECTED IN THE MATERNITY WARD
Skin color: 1 White ( ) 2 Brown ( )　　　3 Black ( )　　4 Yellow ( )　　5 Indigenous ( )
What is your marital status? 1 Married / Stable union ( ) 2 Single ( ) 3 Divorced ( )　　　4 Widowed ( )
Where do you live? 1 Rural area ( )　　　2 Urban area ( )　　　9 Don't know ( )
Did the mother have prenatal care during the child's pregnancy? 1 Yes ( ) 2 No ( ) 9 Don't know ( )
How many consultations have you had?　Consultations 88 - No PN ( ) 99 - Don't know (__________________)
Did you receive advice on breastfeeding during your child's prenatal care? 1 Yes (　　) 　 2 No (　　　) 　 8 No PN (　　　　) 　 9 Don't know　　(　)
Who advised you about breastfeeding during your child's pregnancy? 1 Doctor (　　　 2 Nurse (　　　　) 3 Nursing Technician ( ) 4 CHW ( ) 8 Did not receive guidance ( )　　　9 Doesn't know ( )
Have you had a blood test? 1 Yes ( ) 2 No ( ) 8 No PN ( ) 9 Don't know (　　　　)

If YES, what for:

1. Anemia: 1 Yes (   )   2 No (   )   8 No PN (   )   9 Don't know ( )

2. Syphilis (VDRL): 1 Yes ( ) 2 No ( ) 8 No PN (   )   9 Don't know ( )

3. Diabetes: 1 Yes (   )   2 No (   )   8 No PN (   )   9 Don't know (   )

4. HIV: 1 Yes ( )   2 No ( ) 8 No PN/No test ( ) 9 Don't know ( )

Have you taken a urine test? 1 Yes ( )   2 No ( ) 8 No PN ( )   9 Don't know ( )

Has your breast been examined? 1 Yes ( ) 2 No ( ) 8 No PN ( ) 9 Don't know ( )

Did you have any problems during pregnancy (hypertensive syndrome, gestational diabetes, etc.) 1 Yes (   ), which? 2 No (________________)

How did you give birth? 1 Vaginal ( ) 2 Caesarean ( ) 3 Forceps ( ) 9 Don't know ( )

Were there any problems **with you during childbirth**? 1 Yes ( ), which?

2 No (   ) 99 = Don't know (   )

How long after birth did you breastfeed your child for the first time?   minutes9999   - No breastfeeding (________________)

Did you receive breastfeeding advice at the hospital?

1 Yes (   )   2 No (   )   8 No PN (   )   9 Don't know   (   )

Have you had any breast problems (observe)? 01 Flat or inverted nipples ( ) 02 Nipple fissure ( )
03 Breast engorgement ( ) 04 Obstructed ducts and mastitis ( ) 05 Painful nipples ( ) 00 None ( )

Were you advised on how to treat the breast problem?

01 Yes, by the nurse ( ) 02 Yes, by the nursing technician ( ) 03 Yes, by the doctor ( ) 04 No ( ) 00 No problem ( )

APPENDIX B - Informed consent form
(For mothers aged 18 or over)

Project title: Strategies to strengthen breastfeeding: promoting children's health

Researcher responsible: Luisa Helena de Oliveira Lima

Institution/Department: Federal University of Piauí / Nursing Course / Campus Senador Helvídio Nunes de Barros

Contact telephone number (including collect): (89) 99253737

Participating researchers: Edina Araújo Rodrigues Oliveira

Contact telephone numbers: (89) 99848049

You are being invited to take part in a survey as a volunteer. You need to decide whether you want to take part or not. Please do not rush into making your decision. Read the following carefully and ask the person responsible for the study any questions you may have.

If you agree to take part in the study, please sign at the end of this document, which is in two copies. One copy is yours and the other is for the researcher responsible. If you refuse, you will not be penalized in any way.

My name is Luisa Helena de Oliveira Lima, I'm a nurse and an Adjunct Professor on the Undergraduate Nursing Course at the Federal University of Piauí (UFPI) and I'm currently carrying out research into the factors that influence breastfeeding in the first hour of life in children from Pico, whose data will be collected by nursing and nutrition academics.

There are many factors that can influence breastfeeding. For example, the length of time you have been at school, the weight of the baby, the use of breastfeeding equipment, etc.

pacifier, among others. In this study, I intend to identify the factors that influence breastfeeding in the first hour of life in children from Pico.

If you accept, the academics will fill in a form with you to obtain information about your pregnancy, your delivery, your child's diet and will examine your breasts. In addition, the child will be weighed and its length, head size and the width of its chest and belly will be measured. This physical examination will not pose any risk to the child and discomfort will be kept to a minimum. The study will benefit from greater knowledge of the factors that influence breastfeeding in the first hour of life in children in the municipality of Picos.

You will have the right to withdraw from the research at any time, without any prejudice and/or expense to you.

The data will be presented at scientific events in the health field, respecting the confidentiality of identities.

At any stage of the study, you will have access to the professionals responsible for the research to clarify any doubts you may have.

If you agree to take part in the study, your name and identity will be kept confidential. Unless required by law or at your request, only the researcher, the study team, the independent Ethics Committee and government regulatory agency inspectors (where necessary) will have access to your information to verify the study information.

Consent to the participation of the person as subject

I,

____

,RG

____

, undersigned, agree to participate in the study
Strategies to strengthen breastfeeding: promoting child health, as a subject and I allow my child to participate. I have been sufficiently informed about the information I have read or that has been read to me describing the study Strategies to strengthen breastfeeding: promoting child health. I discussed my decision to take part in this study

____

with the academic. It was made clear to me the purposes of the study, the procedures to be carried out, the discomforts and risks, the guarantees of confidentiality and ongoing clarification.

I have also been informed that my participation and that of my child is free of charge. I voluntarily agree to participate in this study and may withdraw my consent at any time, before or during the study, without penalty or loss of any benefit I may have acquired.

Place and date _______________________Name and signature of subject or guardian:

We witnessed the request for consent, clarifications about the research and the subject's acceptance to participate.

Witnesses (not related to the research team): Name:

ID: _____________ Signature: _______________________________________

Name: ____ RG:

____

Signature: ____

(Only for the researcher responsible for contacting and taking the ICF)

I declare that I have properly and voluntarily obtained the Free and Informed Consent of this research subject or legal representative to participate in this study.

Picos, _____ of __________________201__.

Researcher responsible

Additional notes

If you have any concerns or questions about the ethics of the research, please contact:Research Ethics Committee - UFPI - Campus Universitário Ministro Petronio Portella - Bairro Ininga

Centro de Convivencia L09 e 10 - CEP: 64.049-550 - Teresina - PI

tel.: (86) 3215-5734 - email: cep.ufpi@ufpi.br web: www.ufpi.br/cep

APPENDIX C - Informed consent form

(For mothers under 18)

Project title: Strategies to strengthen breastfeeding: promoting children's health

Researcher responsible: Luisa Helena de Oliveira Lima

Institution/Department: Federal University of Piauí / Nursing Course / Campus Senador Helvídio Nunes de Barros

Contact telephone number (including collect): (89) 99253737 Participating researchers: Edina Araújo Rodrigues Oliveira Contact telephone numbers: (89) 99848049

Your daughter and grandson are being invited to take part in a research project as volunteers. You need to decide whether you want them to take part or not. Please don't rush into making the decision. Please read the following carefully and ask the person responsible for the study any questions you may have. Once you have been informed of the following information, if you agree to your daughter and grandson taking part in the study, please sign at the end of this document, which is in two copies. One copy is yours and the other belongs to the researcher responsible. In the event of refusal, you, your daughter and your grandchild will not be penalized in any way.

My name is Luisa Helena de Oliveira Lima, I'm a nurse and an Adjunct Professor on the Undergraduate Nursing Course at the Federal University of Piauí (UFPI) and I'm currently carrying out research into the factors that influence breastfeeding in the first hour of life in children from Pico, whose data will be collected by nursing and nutrition students.

There are various factors that can influence breastfeeding. For example, the length of time the mother has been at school, the baby's weight, the baby's use of a pacifier, among others. In this study, I intend to identify the factors that influence breastfeeding in the first hour of life in children from Pico.

If you accept, the academics will fill in a form with your daughter to obtain information about her pregnancy, her birth, the feeding of your grandchild and will examine your daughter's breasts. In addition, the child will be weighed and its length, head size and the width of its chest and belly will be measured. This physical examination will not pose any risk to the child and discomfort will be kept to a minimum. The study will benefit from greater knowledge of the factors that influence breastfeeding in the first hour of life in children in the municipality of Picos.

You have the right to withdraw your child and grandchild from the study at any time, without any harm and/or expense to you.

The data will be presented at scientific events in the field of health, respecting the confidentiality of identities.

At any stage of the study, you will have access to the professionals responsible for the research to clarify any doubts you may have.

If you agree to your daughter and grandson participating in the study, their

names and identities will be kept confidential. Unless required by law or at your request, only the researcher, the study team, the independent Ethics Committee and inspectors from government regulatory agencies (when necessary) will have access to your information to verify the study information. Consent of the person to participate as a subject. I, _____________________, RG _____________________,
undersigned, agree to my daughter and grandson participating in the study Strategies to strengthen breastfeeding: promoting child health, as subjects. I have been sufficiently informed about the information I have read or that has been read to me describing the study Strategies to strengthen breastfeeding: promoting child health. I have discussed with the academic my __decision to allow my daughter and grandchild to _____________________take part in this study. It was made clear to me the purposes of the study, the procedures to be carried out, the discomforts and risks, the guarantees of confidentiality and ongoing clarification.

I have also been informed that my daughter and grandson will participate free of charge. I voluntarily agree to participate in this study and may withdraw my consent at any time, before or during the study, without penalty or loss of any benefit I may have acquired. Place and date _____________ Subject's name and signature or responsible: _____________________

We witnessed the request for consent, clarifications about the research and the subject's acceptance to take part.

Witnesses (not connected to the research team): Name:

ID: _________ Signature: _____________________

Name: _____________________ RG: _________

Signature: _____________________

(Only for the researcher responsible for contacting and taking the ICF)

I declare that I have properly and voluntarily obtained the Free and Informed Consent of this research subject or legal representative to participate in this study.

Picos, ____ of ________ 201__ . _____________________

Researcher responsible

Additional notesIf you have any considerations or questions about the ethics of the research, please get in touch:

Research Ethics Committee - UFPI - Campus Universitário Ministro Petronio Portella - Bairro Ininga - Centro de Convivencia L09 e 10 - CEP: 64.049-550 - Teresina - PI tel.: (86) 3215-5734 - email: cep.ufpi@ufpi.br web: www.ufpi.br/cep

APPENDIX D - Informed consent form
(For mothers under 18 years of age)

Project title: Strategies to strengthen breastfeeding: promoting children's health

Researcher responsible: Luisa Helena de Oliveira Lima

Institution/Department: Federal University of Piauí / Nursing Course / Campus Senador Helvídio Nunes de Barros

Contact telephone number (including collect): (89) 99253737

Participating researchers: Edina Araújo Rodrigues Oliveira

Contact telephone numbers: (89) 99848049

You are being invited to take part in a survey as a volunteer. You need to decide whether you want to take part or not. Please do not rush into making your decision. Read the following carefully and ask the study leader any questions you may have.

If you agree to take part in the study, please sign at the end of this document, which is in two copies. One copy is yours and the other belongs to the researcher responsible. If you refuse, you will not be penalized in any way.

My name is Luisa Helena de Oliveira Lima, I'm a nurse and an Adjunct Professor on the Undergraduate Nursing Course at the Federal University of Piauí (UFPI) and I'm currently carrying out research into the factors that influence breastfeeding in the first hour of life in children from Pico, whose data will be collected by nursing and nutrition students.

There are many factors that can influence breastfeeding. For example, the length of time you studied at school, the weight of the baby, the use of a pacifier by the baby, among others. In this study, I intend to identify the factors that influence breastfeeding in the first hour of life in children from Pico.

If you accept, the academics will fill in a form with you to obtain information about your pregnancy, your delivery, your child's diet and will examine your breasts. In addition, the child will be weighed and its length, head size and the width of its chest and belly will be measured. This physical examination will not pose any risk to the child and discomfort will be kept to a minimum. The study will benefit from greater knowledge of the factors that influence breastfeeding in the first hour of life in children in the municipality of Picos.

You will have the right to withdraw from the research at any time, without any prejudice and/or expense to you.

The data will be presented at scientific events in the field of health, respecting the confidentiality of identities.

At any stage of the study, you will have access to the professionals responsible for the research to answer any questions you may have.

If you agree to participate in the study, your name and identity will be kept confidential. Unless required by law or at your request, only the researcher, the study team, the independent Ethics Committee and inspectors from government regulatory agencies (where necessary) will have access to your information to verify the study information.

Consent to the participation of the person as subject

I _________________________________ , the undersigned, agree to to participate in the study Strategies to strengthen breastfeeding: promoting children's health, as a subject and I allow my child to participate. I have been sufficiently informed about the information I have read or that has been read to me describing the study Strategies to strengthen breastfeeding: promoting child health. I have discussed with the academic ____
about my decision to take part in this study. It was made clear to me the purposes of the study, the procedures to be carried out, the discomforts and risks, the guarantees of confidentiality and ongoing clarification.

I have also been informed that my participation and that of my child is free of charge. I voluntarily agree to participate in this study and may withdraw my consent at any time, before or during the study, without penalty or loss of any benefit I may have acquired.

Place and date Subject's name and signature:

       We witnessed the request for consent, clarifications about the research and the subject's acceptance to participate.

Witnesses (not related to the research team):Name:

ID: _________ Signature: ____

Name: ____RG:

____

Signature: _________________________________

(Only for the researcher responsible for contacting and taking the consent form)

I declare that I have properly and voluntarily obtained the Free and Informed Consent of this research subject or legal representative to participate in this study.

Picos, ____ of _________ 201__ .

       Researcher responsible

Additional notes

If you have any considerations or questions about the ethics of the research, please get in touch:

Research Ethics Committee - UFPI - Campus Universitário Ministro Petronio Portella - Bairro Ininga - Centro de Convivencia L09 e 10 - CEP: 64.049-550 - Teresina - PI tel.: (86) 3215-5734 - email: cep.ufpi@ufpi.br web: www.ufpi.br/ce

ANNEX
ANNEX A - Research Ethics Committee approval report

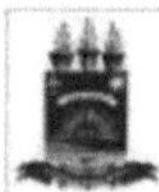 UNIVERSIDADE FEDERAL DO PIAUÍ - UFPI 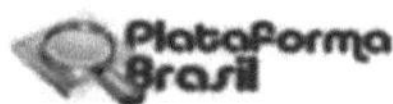

PARECER CONSUBSTANCIADO DO CEP

DADOS DO PROJETO DE PESQUISA

Título da Pesquisa: Fatores associados à amamentação na primeira hora de vida em crianças picoenses: um estudo transversal
Pesquisador: LUISA HELENA DE OLIVEIRA LIMA
Área Temática:
Versão: 2
CAAE: 46039015.6.0000.5214
Instituição Proponente: Universidade Federal do Piauí - UFPI
Patrocinador Principal: Financiamento Próprio

DADOS DO PARECER

Número do Parecer: 1.144.279
Data da Relatoria: 31/07/2015

Apresentação do Projeto:
Estudo de natureza descritiva do tipo transversal, pois serão investigados os fatores associados à amamentação na primeira hora de vida em crianças picoenses. O estudo será realizado em um hospital público de referência do município de Picos – PI.
A população será composta por todas as crianças nascidas vivas no período de junho de 2015 a maio de 2016. Para estimativa do tamanho da população, utilizou-se o número de nascidos vivos no referido hospital no ano de 2013, totalizando 924 nascidos vivos. A amostra será censitária, pois trabalharemos com todos os nascidos vivos. Os participantes serão selecionados de forma consecutiva, à medida que forem nascendo, e que preencherem os critérios de elegibilidade. Para participar as crianças e mães terão que atender os seguintes critérios de inclusão: - criança nascida viva, no período da coleta (junho de 2015 a maio de 2016); - criança cujo responsável aceite participar da pesquisa e assine o termo de consentimento livre e esclarecido. Serão considerados critérios de exclusão: - RN com muito baixo peso ao nascer inferior a 1.500g ou com idade gestacional (método Capurro) menor que 32 semanas, que impossibilite a permanência em alojamento conjunto; - óbito fetal ou neonatal precoce; - óbito materno; - destino da puérpera – unidade semiintensiva; - mãe com

Endereço: Campus Universitário Ministro Petronio Portella - Pró-Reitoria de Pesquisa
Bairro: Ininga   CEP: 64.049-550
UF: PI   Município: TERESINA
Telefone: (86)3237-2332   Fax: (86)3237-2332   E-mail: cep.ufpi@ufpi.edu.br

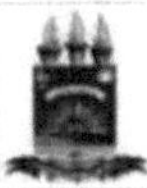 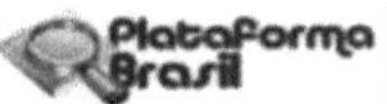

UNIVERSIDADE FEDERAL DO PIAUÍ - UFPI

sorologia positiva para HIV no pré-natal registrada em prontuário. Para coletar os dados será utilizado um formulário (apêndice C) adaptado de outros estudos (BOCCOLINI et al., 2011; CAMINHA et al., 2010). O formulário contém informações sobre identificação da criança, antropometria ao nascimento, dados sobre a gravidez e pré-natal da mãe, condições do parto e aleitamento materno no primeiro dia de vida. Este formulário será preenchido com a mãe ainda na maternidade.

Objetivo da Pesquisa:

Objetivo Primário:

Investigar os fatores associados à amamentação na primeira hora de vida em crianças picoenses

Objetivo Secundário:

Traçar o perfil socioeconômico e sanitário das crianças e mães pesquisadas ;Identificar a prevalência de aleitamento materno (AM) e de aleitamento materno exclusivo (AMEX) na primeira hora de vida na população estudada;Descrever os fatores de proteção ao AM na primeira hora de vida na população estudada;Levantar as dificuldades para desenvolvimento do AM e AMEX na primeira hora de vida na população pesquisada;Analisar a influência do tipo de parto para o desenvolvimento da amamentação na primeira hora de vida;Verificar a influência do acompanhamento pré-natal para o desenvolvimento da amamentação na primeira hora de vida.

Avaliação dos Riscos e Benefícios:

"Riscos:

Este exame físico não trará risco para a criança e o desconforto será o mínimo possível. Tentaremos reduzir este desconforto fazendo o exame físico de maneira delicada e utilizando as técnicas adequadas.

Benefícios:

O estudo trará como benefício um maior conhecimento dos os fatores que influenciam no aleitamento materno na primeira hora de vida em crianças no município de Picos."

Comentários e Considerações sobre a Pesquisa:

Pesquisa de tema relevante para a saúde da criança, considerando que a amamentação está associada a risco reduzido de várias infecções neonatais, incluindo infecções gastrintestinais, infecções diarreicas, e infecções do tipo de extra-intestinais.

Endereço: Campus Universitário Ministro Petronio Portella - Pró-Reitoria de Pesquisa
Bairro: Ininga   CEP: 64.049-550
UF: PI   Município: TERESINA
Telefone: (86)3237-2332   Fax: (86)3237-2332   E-mail: cep.ufpi@ufpi.edu.br

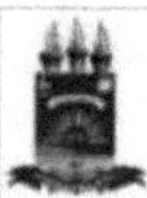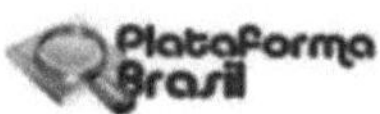

Continuação do Parecer: 1.144.2/9

Considerações sobre os Termos de apresentação obrigatória:
Todos os termos foram apresentados corretamente.

Recomendações:
Sem recomendações.

Conclusões ou Pendências e Lista de Inadequações:
Atendidas as pendências o projeto encontra-se apto a ser desenvolvido do pontos de vista ético.

Situação do Parecer:
Aprovado

Necessita Apreciação da CONEP:
Não

Considerações Finais a critério do CEP:
O CEP aguarda o envio dos relatórios parciais e final da pesquisa.

TERESINA, 09 de Julho de 2015

Assinado por:
Adrianna de Alencar Setubal Santos
(Coordenador)

Endereço: Campus Universitário Ministro Petronio Portella - Pró-Reitoria de Pesquisa
Bairro: Ininga   CEP: 64.049-560
UF: PI   Município: TERESINA
Telefone: (86)3237-2332   Fax: (86)3237-2332   E-mail: cep.ufpi@ufpi.edu.br

Página 22 de 43

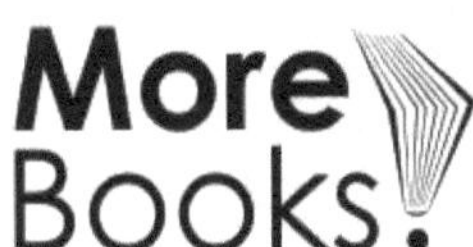

More
Books!

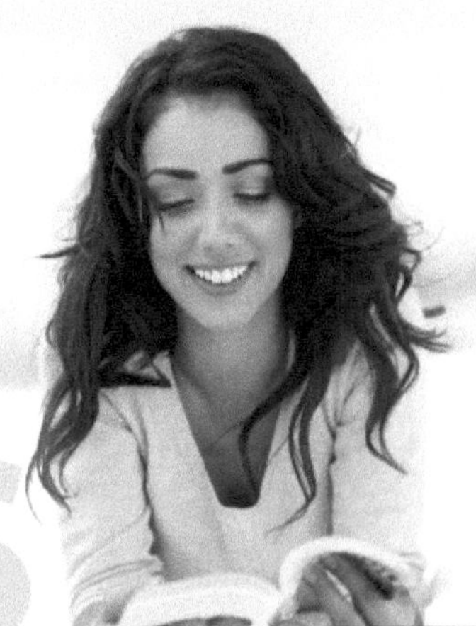

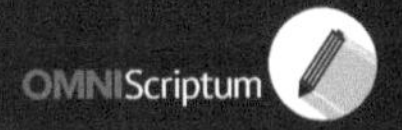

info@omniscriptum.com
www.omniscriptum.com
OMNIScriptum

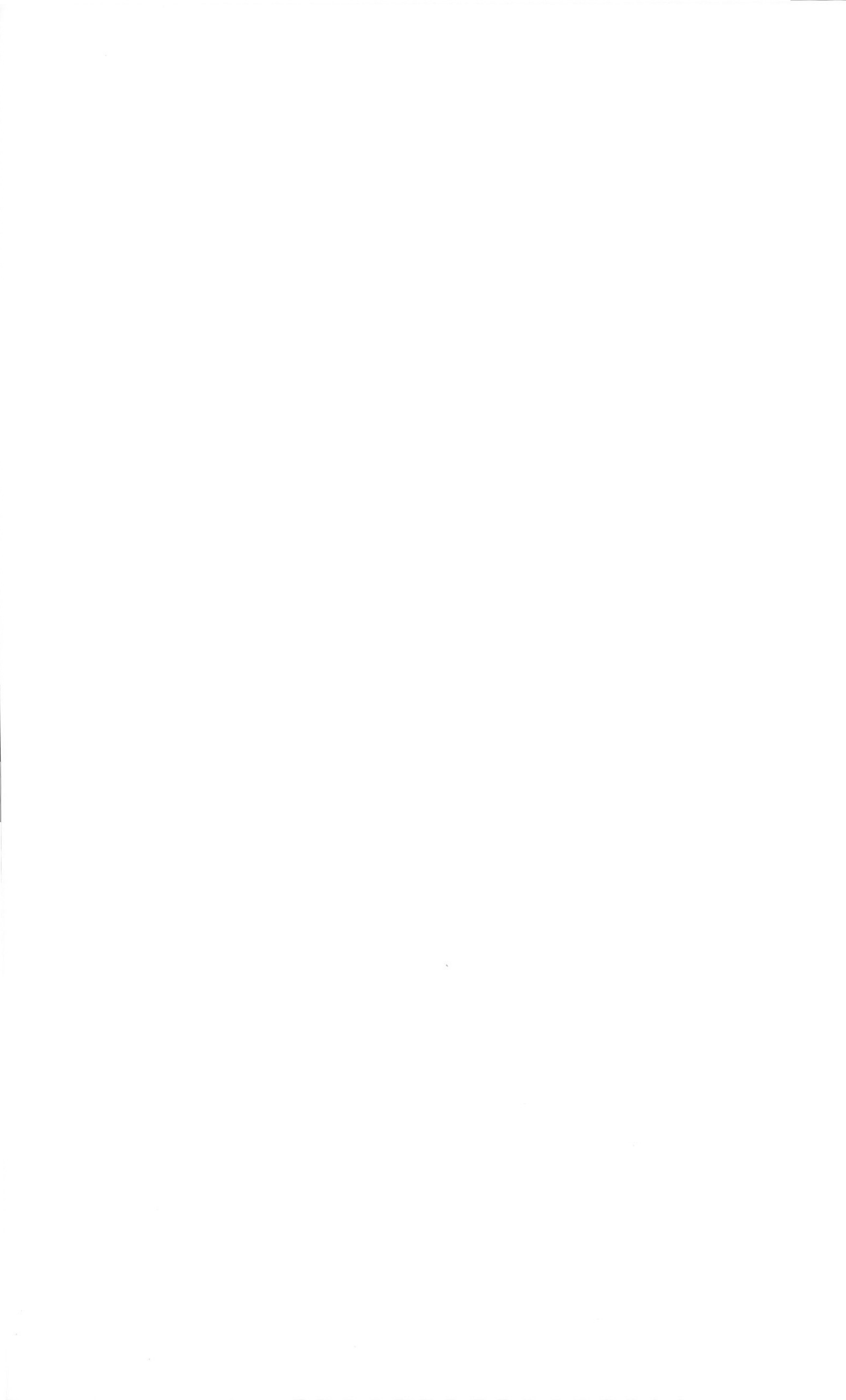

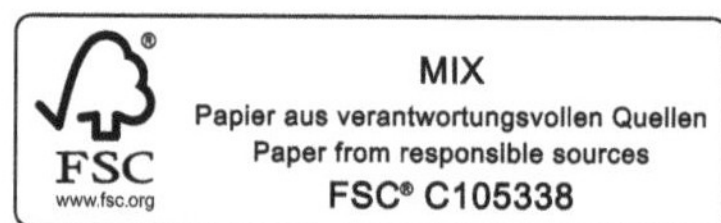

Printed by Books on Demand GmbH, Norderstedt / Germany